GOING LOCAL

Increasingly social workers and social care professionals have to develop effective community and neighbourhood-based approaches for delivering their services. The pressure for this has arisen partly from government, which is directing services to engage fully with local communities, and partly from local people themselves who want, and expect, a greater say in shaping the services they receive.

Going Local is written for students and practitioners of all kinds, including those working with older people, children and families, and young people. The volume explains how to develop approaches to working in communities and neighbourhoods, engage with users and their locality, and contribute to strengthening local communities. Topics discussed include:

- Why social work services need to 'go local'
- The major concepts, perspectives and policies underpinning work in communities and neighbourhoods
- How to gather information about a specific neighbourhood
- How to maximise the involvement of local people in shaping services
- How to develop effective partnerships with local organisations
- Specific approaches to delivering neighbourhood and community services for older people, children and families and young people
- The role of practitioners in overcoming cultural and ethnic divisions within communities.

With activities, chapter overviews and key points summarised in each chapter, this textbook will appeal to social work students and social care professionals concerned with neighbourhood and community-based services. It is also essential reading for a wide range of practitioners in local authorities and voluntary and non-profit organisations as well as youth workers, community development practitioners and the probation service.

John Pierson was formerly Senior Lecturer in social work and applied social studies at Staffordshire University. He now works as a policy analyst and is a visiting lecturer at the Creative Communities Unit at Staffordshire University, UK.

the social work skills series

published in association with *Community Care*

series editor: Terry Philpot

the social work skills series

- builds practice skills step by step

- places practice in its policy context

- relates practice to relevant research

- provides a secure base for professional development

This new, skills-based series has been developed by Routledge and *Community Care* working together in partnership to meet the changing needs of today's students and practitioners in the broad field of social care. Written by experienced practitioners and teachers with a commitment to passing on their knowledge to the next generation, each text in the series features: *learning objectives; case examples; activities to test knowledge and understanding; summaries of key learning points; key references; suggestions for further reading.*

Also available in the series:

Commissioning and Purchasing
Terry Bamford
Former Chair of the British Association of
Social Workers and Executive Director
of Housing and Social Services, Royal
Borough of Kensington and Chelsea.

Managing Aggression
Ray Braithwaite
Consultant and trainer in managing
aggression at work. Lead trainer and
speaker in the 'No Fear' campaign.

Tackling Social Exclusion
John Pierson
Senior Lecturer at the Institute of Social
Work and Applied Social Studies at the
University of Staffordshire.

Safeguarding Children and Young People
Corinne May-Chahal and Stella Coleman
Professor of Applied Social Science at
Lancaster University.
Senior Lecturer in Social Work at the
University of Central Lancashire.

The Task-Centred Book
Mark Doel and Peter Marsh
Research Professor of Social Work at
Sheffield Hallam University.
Professor of Child and Family Welfare,
University of Sheffield.

Using Groupwork
Mark Doel
Research Professor of Social Work at
Sheffield Hallam University.

Practising Welfare Rights
Neil Bateman
Author, trainer and consultant specialising
in welfare rights and social policy issues

GOING LOCAL

Working in communities and neighbourhoods

John Pierson

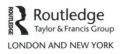
Routledge
Taylor & Francis Group

LONDON AND NEW YORK

communitycare

First published 2008
by Routledge
2 Park Square, Milton Park, Abingdon, Oxon OX14 4RN

Simultaneously published in the USA and Canada
by Routledge
270 Madison Ave, New York, NY 10016

Routledge is an imprint of the Taylor & Francis Group, an informa business

© 2008 John Pierson

Typeset in Sabon
by Keystroke, High Street, Tettenhall, Wolverhampton
Printed and bound in Great Britain
by TJ International Ltd, Padstow, Cornwall

British Library Cataloguing in Publication Data
A catalogue record for this book is available from the British Library

Library of Congress Cataloging in Publication Data
Pierson, John, 1944–
Going local : working in communities and neighbourhoods / John Pierson.
p. cm. – (Social work skills series)
Includes bibliographical references and index.
ISBN 978–0–415–34780–8 (hardback) – ISBN 978–0–415–32840–1 (pbk.)
1. Community-based social services. 2. Community development.
3. Community organization. I. Title.
HV41.P547 2007
361.2′5–dc22
2007001060

ISBN10: 0–415–34780–7 (hbk)
ISBN10: 0–415–32840–3 (pbk)
ISBN10: 0–203–37043–0 (ebk)

ISBN13: 978–0–415–34780–8 (hbk)
ISBN13: 978–0–415–32840–1 (pbk)
ISBN13: 978–0–203–37043–8 (ebk)

To Martin Thomas,
a steadfast friend, colleague and enabler
with gratitude

CONTENTS

FIGURES

ACTIVITIES

BOXES

CASE STUDIES

ACKNOWLEDGEMENTS

I would like to thank the following for many helpful conversations, ideas, and information which I readily took advantage of in the preparation of this book:

Fiona Green, Val Nicholls of Sure Start Blurton, Liz Reynolds of Stoke-on-Trent Lifelong Learning and Education, Dr Jacqueline Barnes of Birkbeck College, University of London, Sheila Brooke of Blacon Neighbourhood Management Pathfinder, Neil Jameson of the Citizens' Organising Foundation, Faraz Yousufzai of Working Links, Birmingham, Kirk Knoden of Youngstown Ohio Gamaliel, Sajida Madni of Birmingham Citizens, Penny Vincent of Stoke-on-Trent City Council, Bernard Bester, District Partnership Office of Staffordshire County Council, Steve Johnston of Stoke City Council Knowledge Management Unit, Barbara Emadi-Coffin and Mark Webster of the Creative Communities Unit, Staffordshire University, Bob MacLaren, head of Children's Services, Wrexham Social Services, Clare Worley of Manchester Metropolitan University, Santokh Gill of the Bradford Young People's Research Project, and Eric Beak, Sally Sharp and the volunteers and young people at Malpas Young Persons' Centre.

I would like to thank Frank Pierson, lead organiser for the Industrial Areas Foundation in the US for many discussions on citizen action and for the idea of 'the church of accidents'. I am especially grateful to Paul Boylan, Manager of the Blacon Neighbourhood Management Pathfinder, who is both an outstanding servant for the public good and a ready source of innovative ideas and projects of national importance.

I thank the following publishers for permission to use material from their publications: The Joseph Rowntree Foundation for *Benchmarking Community Participation* by Wilson and Wilde, Taylor and Francis for an article by Clare Wenger in *Aging and Mental Health*, New Society Press for *The Mediator's Handbook* by Beer and Stief and *Facilitator's Guide to Participatory Decision-making*, Blacon Neighbourhood Management Pathfinder for the *Community Engagement Checklist*, Seven Locks Press for *Organizing for Social Change*, the Policy Press for *Managing Community Practice* by Banks *et al.*, Jane Carrier for *Older People: The New Agenda*, Jessica Kingsley Publishers for *Adolescence: Assessing and Promoting Resilience* by Daniel and Wassell and Barnardos for *The Missing Side of the Triangle*.

Every effort has been made to contact and acknowledge copyright owners, but the author and publishers would be pleased to have any errors or omissions brought to their attention so that corrections may be published at a later printing.

INTRODUCTION

All good social work is local. As a profession its origins lie in intensive face-to-face work in the tightly drawn urban slums of mid and late nineteenth century Britain when, through a variety of approaches and ideologies, the first systematic efforts were made to improve the level of well-being of the urban poor. This connection with neighbourhoods, particularly disadvantaged neighbourhoods, must remain a focus of work today. Without a commitment to acting as a major agent in the effort to establish higher levels of well-being in the communities and neighbourhoods of Britain, one of the main missions of social work dries up and loses its energy and vision. Only by working with people *and* the environment in which they live does social work roll back the effects of poverty, give voice to the voiceless and pursue that vision of social justice which forms its historic mission.

Yet this link with community and neighbourhood has often been overshadowed by other professional concerns, and in particular, for much of the twentieth century, submerged beneath a view that primarily an individual should be understood as a psychological animal first and a social animal second (Specht and Courtney 1994). This had the effect of filtering massive social problems, actually arising from the structure of inequality and exploitation of urban neighbourhoods, through the lens of the frailties and poor choices of individuals and families. According to this perspective, solutions lay in reforming the habits and behaviour of individuals. As this perspective took hold in professional thinking it cut off other possible courses of practitioner activity.

This perspective is no longer sustainable. Our fast growing knowledge of the complexity of the interaction between a person and their environment makes the idea of a bright line between what pertains to the individual and family (the old province of social work) and what pertains to social structure (conceded by social work to the political domain) obsolete. There are now strands of practice developing which in effect ask the practitioner to work back and forth between individuals and families on the one hand and the environment that impinges, then constrains and oppresses – or supports and facilitates – their life chances on the other.

This volume seeks to recover and underscore the importance of neighbourhoods and communities as a principal arena of practice. It aims to rebalance social work's own view of itself, its tasks and roles in the direction of greater interest and involvement in users' local environment. This does not mean sacrificing the long-standing professional commitment to 'the person' nor the uniqueness of each individual and family. Rather it argues that to undertake this work more effectively social work and social care must directly promote those elements in neighbourhoods and communities that foster well-being and human flourishing. In short, social work and social care require the capacity both to work with 'people' *and* with 'place'.

The volume is written with the conviction that, despite its rich tradition of community focus, social work has forgotten those skills associated with that tradition and has not developed sufficiently the new skills and knowledge now required for effective work in localities. Attitudes on the part of practitioners and managers alike seemed to say: 'Community? We are not community workers, we work with individuals and their families' or 'neighbourhood well-being? We would like to help but we are too busy putting out fires and besides there's no money to do anything else'.

The argument of this volume seeks to move beyond this artificial and unnecessary division. It does not offer a single path for practitioners to pursue, still less a single recipe for embedding services in communities and neighbourhoods. The aim is broad: to show how social work can engage communities and neighbourhoods more purpose-fully. As is made clear over the following chapters, this requires no more than dedication to three broad, flexible themes:

- developing effective relationships with local people
- utilising local knowledge
- viewing social problems holistically.

In a phrase, 'going local' presents practitioners with ways to cease 'seeing like a state' (Scott 1998) and to work with citizens and other mainstream and community service providers to build the capacity of neighbourhoods to tackle social problems on their own.

A short explanation of the terms 'social work', 'social worker' and 'social care' as used in this volume is necessary. In its broadest usage social work as a field of endeavour has expanded enormously but also fragmented into a range of posts, tasks and responsibilities that too often do not even use the phrase 'social work' to describe those activities. Nonetheless, because of its historical associations and its expansiveness the term is still preferred to the now more ubiquitous 'social care worker', which for all its ubiquity is so indistinct as to be meaningless. This volume uses the phrase 'social work' in its broadest sense covering a wide range of activities, roles and respon-sibilities across the voluntary, private and public sectors. It embraces local authority social workers, youth workers, care managers, youth justice workers, probation officers, school-based social workers, inclusion officers, those tackling anti-social behaviour, advice workers, family support workers, early years workers, child care workers, resi-dential care staff and community development officers. It includes service 'navigators' and brokers working with older people and disabled people in social care, as well as those in community drug action teams or assertive outreach for people with mental health problems. It includes those working in domestic violence projects, helping asylum seekers and refugees settle in to a new town, or helping a community resolve its policy towards sex workers. Social work is a big tent and this volume is aimed at all those who deliver services to children, families, vulnerable adults and older people and who either have a community or neighbourhood dimension to their work or are interested in exploring the possibilities offered by such work. Occasionally the phrase 'social work and social care' is used in the volume simply to underscore the broad reference to a multiplicity of posts and roles.

Clearly 'going local' is not the only agenda for contemporary social work and social care – there are others including some that conflict directly with it. For example, protecting and safeguarding children and families will continue to suck resources away from the provision of community-based early intervention and preventative support services. In relation to services for young people the Respect agenda and the crackdown on anti-social behaviour may clash with the provision of support for young people in transition to adulthood. The white paper on social care (Department of Health (DoH) 2006a) began to reposition the health and social care services towards prevention and tackling the inequalities of provision, but that practice also remains captured by a strong tilt towards national health and medical systems jeopardising the strengths, perspectives and focus on exclusion that social work and its allied professions bring when tackling difficult social problems.

Going local, then, cannot be reduced to a simple imperative such as 'get acquainted with your neighbourhood', or adding a neighbourhood veneer to practice. But neither should it be based on asking social workers to become something they cannot possibly be. This volume is not about turning social workers into community workers – they are too embedded in specific roles and mandated functions for that. (In any case the free-floating community worker who comes into a neighbourhood to help groups organise and give voice to problems that beset them is a disappearing breed.) But the volume lays out what might be called 'cross-over practice', a practice that is more flexible and wide ranging and prepared to intervene in neighbourhood and community structures, thus going beyond formal remits of the past. Social workers and social care workers are already doing more community-oriented work now than they might realise. One of the objectives of the book is to see this work more accurately for what it is and to be clear when practitioners are engaging at a community or neighbourhood level. It asks practitioners to look at a wider theatre for operation, adopt a wider sense of the potential for collaboration and above all a far stronger commitment to the kinds of services that local citizens* are calling for. The volume is about encouraging a *direction*, about practitioners pressing ahead into areas that are logical extensions of their work, and developing the additional skills and approaches that will make this happen.

THE STRUCTURE OF THE BOOK

The aim of this volume is to move with the wider tide: to explain the pressures and trends towards greater engagement with locality and to ensure that the connection between social work and the communities and neighbourhoods it serves will only strengthen in the future.

The following chapters are intended to provide further exploration of what a local, neighbourhood practice is. Chapter 1 explains why neighbourhoods are so critical in the life of service users and establishes the case for incorporating neighbourhood- and community-level interventions in the practice repertoire. Chapter 2 gets the reader started in thinking about a community-oriented practice and lays out four pillars of that

---

* The term 'citizen' is used here in its global meaning as a bearer of rights, capabilities and powers and *not* simply the passport holder from a particular nation. See Edwards and Gaventa 2000.

work. Chapter 3 presents the cornerstones for a holistic service to neighbourhoods and communities through joined-up practice and the formation of local alliances and partnerships. It also examines the power of social networks to deliver outcomes for both practitioners and users. Chapter 4 brings together some of the skills, tools and approaches needed to engage with communities and neighbourhoods. It specifically looks at setting up neighbourhood forums and techniques for facilitation and running meetings.

The remaining chapters deal with specific service areas, drawing out those approaches that already have a community or neighbourhood remit as well as those approaches that can be crafted for greater impact on neighbourhood-wide structures and attitudes. Chapter 5 deals with services for children and families in neighbourhoods; Chapter 6 looks at community safety and improving the lives of young people while responding to calls to tackle anti-social behaviour and community-based justice; Chapter 7 addresses the links between the promotion of well-being and dignity for older people while they remain in their communities of choice. Each of these chapters considers how neighbourhood practice can emerge from social work processes such as assessment or commissioning support services.

Chapter 8 examines the seriousness of the ethnic and religious divisions in Britain's urban neighbourhoods and examines the approaches and principles that social work and social care can follow in pursuing goals of mutual toleration and improved community well-being. In the early 1900s the African American W. E. B. DuBois said, 'the problem of the twentieth century is the colour line'. The challenge of the twenty-first century is the conciliation of different, even opposing, moral, religious and cultural forces. As with challenging racism, so in this endeavour does social work have a key role to play. Chapter 9 concludes the volume by discussing some of the points raised in the activities throughout the book.

CHAPTER 1

WORKING IN COMMUNITIES AND NEIGHBOURHOODS

By the end of this chapter you should:

- Understand why neighbourhoods and communities are essential arenas for practice

- Be familiar with definitions of 'neighbourhood' and 'community'

- Know the research findings on 'neighbourhood effects' – how neighbourhoods impact on service outcomes and people's well-being

- Be familiar with the major community and neighbourhood focus of government policies for public services

- Begin to think how social work and social care practice can adapt in order to engage communities and neighbourhoods.

DEFINING 'NEIGHBOURHOOD' AND 'COMMUNITY'

Throughout this volume the terms 'neighbourhood' and 'community' are sometimes used together, sometimes separately. The reason for this is partly pragmatic: both terms are widely used in policy documents issued by government and by research and social care practitioners. Although there are differences in emphasis and attributes at one level both concepts convey the same idea – that of a spatial environment, a bounded locality in which people may *or may not* feel some sense of affinity, attachment and recognition. Neither term is used in this volume in ways that assume the existence of rosy, street-level relationships in which neighbours are in and out of each other's homes bringing good cheer and support. But as we shall see, while contemporary use of the terms 'neighbourhoods' and 'communities' no longer evokes an earlier golden age that itself was overblown, the terms do have qualities and assets as spatial entities that social workers need to focus more clearly on: social networks, housing environments, institutions such as schools and places of worship, and community organisations.

'Neighbourhood'

For most people 'the neighbourhood' means the small area immediately around where they live, while 'neighbours' are those who live in households nearby with whom social relations, by no means always close, are generally based on face-to-face contact. But in government policy and practitioner thinking about spatial environments 'neighbourhood' is generally used to denote far larger geographical areas than is commonly understood by most of us. There are several rules of thumb used to define neighbourhoods in this larger sense. Some of these are: an area mapped out by how far a person can walk in any direction in 15 minutes; an area defined by landmarks as recognised by most residents who live near them; common boundaries established by roads or housing tenure; political ward boundaries or areas with an historical identity such as parishes. These in turn often reflect population clusters and natural boundary points, street patterns, housing tenures, social networks – all important constituents of neighbourhood definition. The neighbourhoods referred to in this volume are often defined by a mixture of these and may embrace 3,000 or so households with perhaps as many as 6,000 residents.

Local communities were defined by urban sociologists early in the twentieth century, particularly in the US, as 'natural areas' that developed as a result of competition between businesses for land use and between population groups for affordable housing. A neighbourhood was a subsection of this – 'a collection of both people and institutions occupying a spatially defined area influenced by ecological, cultural and sometimes political forces' (Park 1916 cited by Sampson and Gannon-Rowley 2002: 445). Suttles expanded Park's definition to include imposed boundaries and argued that a local community is not a single entity but rather a hierarchy of progressively more inclusive residential groupings, within which neighbourhoods sit (Suttles 1972 cited by Sampson and Gannon-Rowley: 445).

BOX 1.1: DEFINITION OF 'NEIGHBOURHOOD' AND 'COMMUNITY'

Neighbourhoods 'are an ecological unit that are nested within successively larger communities. There is no one neighbourhood, but many neighbourhoods that vary in size and complexity depending on the social phenomenon of interest and the ecological structure of the larger community. This idea of embeddedness [emphasises] that the local neighbourhood is integrally linked to, and dependent on, a larger whole. For these reasons, one can think of residential neighbourhoods as a "mosaic of overlapping boundaries . . .".

(Sampson 1999: 248)

'Communities can be defined as a group of people sharing values and institutions; specifically, some *social meaning* as well as some organisational structure must connect the individuals to the community. One important component of a community is that it has a sphere that provides a method for production, distribution and consumption of goods and services'.

(Bracht 1999: 31)

'Community'

The concept of 'community' has an even more complicated set of meanings; indeed, the concept of 'neighbourhood' evolved in policy parlance partly to replace the difficulties that the ubiquitous use of 'community' presented. As a term, 'community' emerged very much in opposition to 'society'. It began to be used in something like the way we know it in the nineteenth century, when it came to signify the closer interpersonal relationships that were thought to exist between people in localities. It stood for the informal bonds and connections existing between people in opposition to the kinds of impersonal, alienated, instrumental relationships that characterised mass industrial society.

Critics of 'community' over the last thirty years have sought principally to demystify the concept and to ensure that the sense of togetherness that the word seemed to imply is submitted to careful analysis. An earlier generation of community studies had built up sociological models in which local working class residents shared the burdens and pleasures of living in close-knit terraced streets or mining towns and responded to the rhythms of the mass industrial age: the factory whistle, chapel, wakes, friendly societies and informal support networks among extended families and friends (see for example Young and Willmott 1963). Geographic proximity or locality was the overarching criterion, marking out communities as varied as the East End of London, middle class suburbs, working class districts of manufacturing towns, council housing estates, mining villages. All were relatively homogenous in ethnic and social class make-up with residents holding similar values regarding faith, individual behaviour, family norms and even political views.

Much contemporary analysis of community has moved in the other direction, arguing that there is no such thing as 'the community' in the sense of a single community of people occupying a single geographical space. To speak of such is to privilege the customs and values of a dominant group and to pretend that this one set of values, perspectives and opinions represents the views of all groups within that geographical area. Rather, this critique runs, there are many communities within any given geographical space, each based on different values, different ways of looking at life, and different definitions of well-being. Communities may be formed for example around faith, ethnicity, language, culture or more particularly around disability, sexual orientation and age.

There are also critics who argue that the very fabric of community is weakening. The diversity and mobility of resident populations, the thinning of social networks, the demise of the extended family and the decline in volunteerism have undermined all community orientations, making any policy and practice based on a community focus difficult to sustain. This critique is largely associated with postmodernist thinkers and sociologists who argue that an age of total individualism is upon us in which all social connection is suffering (Beck 1992; Bauman 2001). There are also important commentators who argue that it is supremely unfair and counterproductive to base an entire social policy on asking local 'communities' to tackle huge social problems such as exclusion or lack of public safety from their own eroded local resources (Rose 2000).

Other observers prefer to point to *communities of interest*, which may be locality based but may also exist across large distances. Communities of interest are the result of ties and networks across space and time. They consist of people who have one or more elements of life in common, whether tasks and responsibilities, values, politics, sexuality or faith. Virtually any common commitment or motivation can link some people with others and provide the basis for a community of interest. Churches and mosques are good examples: their members may be drawn from the immediate area in which they are located but equally they may be called from across a large metropolitan or even regional district.

Criticism of 'community' can go too far. Geographical communities and neighbourhoods are *more* than simply geographical space. They contain institutions such as schools, pre-school care and education sites, churches, mosques and synagogues, shops, health centres, local offices, libraries, sports facilities, public transport and community centres. Residents in any given area do live in proximity to each other and will have some sort of relationship, whether supportive, indifferent or even antagonistic. Geographical communities generate associations of many different kinds – horticultural clubs, tenants' and residents' groups, football teams, PTAs and support groups. They embrace a range of activities: low-cost day centres, support groups for shared problems, after-school clubs, breakfast clubs, youth centres. They also embrace social networks and relationships between people.

As with neighbourhoods, there are boundaries to geographical communities recognised by those who live there, and some public acceptance of common coherence. In practice a community's boundaries often simply follow the local authority ward boundaries, but the logic of street patterns and prevalent face-to-face social networks, including consumer patterns, also count (Morenoff *et al.* 2001: 420).

In the wake of the literature on what he describes as 'community lost, community saved and community liberated', Sampson (1999) extends the idea of 'the community of limited liability'. He acknowledges that for many of our deeply personal relationships, as well as those at work, we in the developed world are far less tied to the geographical community in which we live. Nevertheless the concept of community remains essential as a site for the realisation of common values in support of social goods, including public safety, norms of civility and mutual trust, voluntary associations and collective socialisation of the young. Geographical communities are also the place where the inequalities in economic resources and social-structural resources are located and sharply evident. Such resources, particularly income, housing stock and educational attainment are distributed unequally across spatial areas and exert particular pressures on those who do not have access to them (Sampson 1999).

WHY WORKING WITH COMMUNITIES AND NEIGHBOURHOODS IS IMPORTANT

The proliferation in community- and neighbourhood-based services since the end of the 1990s has been remarkable. Both in policy and in service initiatives the emphasis has been to focus services and practitioner energy on localities in order to provide broadly supportive, locally based integrated services to whole groups of local people. Government has had much to do with this trend. It has underscored the need for people to assume greater responsibility for the fate of their own neighbourhood and called for increased levels of participation and involvement in community services, whether schools, social care or care of young children. To back this up it launched powerful neighbourhood-based programmes such as Sure Start, neighbourhood management schemes and Health Action Zones, which directed significant resources into localities that provided many avenues for the involvement of local people.

Funding for neighbourhood services

Looked at from the neighbourhood's point of view the mainstream services spend, in the course of a single year, huge sums of money in providing local services. In an average neighbourhood of some 6,000 households those mainstream services such as health, social services, education, police and housing may spend around £60 million pounds annually. But in terms of visible impact on the quality of services or on the quality of life in that neighbourhood, the outcome of that expenditure is often negligible from residents' point of view. Historically the mainstream services, such as housing, education, social care and police, had little motivation to change direction. These 'service silos' – so called because their stolid, immobile structures are not unlike the tall grain silos found on farms which stand on their own without the capacity to communicate among themselves – tended to view their own services as inherently positive for the community, believing eventually that they would resolve the 'wicked issues' of exclusion, loss of dignity, lack of economic opportunity and unsafe streets. But this was based on a 'bird's-eye' view of community, a perspective taken from high above the streets and homes of residents, and not on local knowledge. At street level the intensity of these problems feels very different, while local services present a picture of anarchy without clear lines of who is responsible for what or who to turn to in order to begin solving these problems.*

Accessibility

Community-based services, then, have often been developed in response to service fragmentation and gaps created by decades of practice based on the birds-eye view. In general, community-based services are more accessible and strive to resolve problems

---

* I am indebted to Paul Boylan of the Neighbourhood Management Pathfinder in Blacon Chester for this point.

as defined by local people. They are available through schools, local offices, well-known community institutions such as churches or mosques, health clinics or in a person's home. They are delivered by personnel, professional and volunteer, that know the area and some of its people. As a rule they do not involve a compromise of personal dignity or dramatic loss of autonomy and are aimed, usually, at whole groups of local people sharing common needs or aspiring to reach common goals.

'NEIGHBOURHOOD EFFECTS': WHAT THE RESEARCH TELLS US

One of the principal drivers for going local with services is our greater understanding of how neighbourhood environments impact on the lives of the people who live there. We now have compelling evidence which shows that where a person lives profoundly affects their life chances and opportunities. Neighbourhoods do matter for the people who live in them. The differences between neighbourhoods, in terms of institutional resources, patterns of social organisation and networks, levels of community safety, quality of physical environment and levels of trust, either support or undermine how people are able to overcome difficulties and develop resilience (Briggs 2002).

In general the concept of 'neighbourhood effects' refers to the powerful environmental impact that living in a particular area has on the health, well-being and life course of individuals who live in that area. One authority summarises it this way: 'Put simply neighbourhood effects occur when geographical location matters over and above personal characteristics'; that is, the extent to which the environment has an impact on service users' life chances and well-being (Overman 2002: 117).

William Wilson's classic study *The Truly Disadvantaged* (Wilson 1987) first outlined the structural dimensions of those neighbourhoods where a high concentration of low-income people live, the ghettos of Chicago, and how this geographic isolation of the poor, from services, jobs, education and labour markets shaped the behaviour of all the residents living there. Wilson discovered that the structure of forces in these neighbourhoods – such as the discrimination by employers towards residents, the total lack of investment, the lack of jobs and job opportunities, the poor levels of services in health and education, the social isolation and lack of transport, the 'redlining' by mortgage companies (the informal practice of estate agents which stops mortgage lending in specific low income areas) – narrowed individual choices and undermined residents' lives at every turn regardless of individual character and behaviour.

Such deprivation, Wilson noted, especially impacts on unskilled young men who encounter so many barriers to the labour market that they adapt to a different, often criminal lifestyle. They fail to acquire skills needed in the labour market, they lose the sense of personal discipline needed to obtain and hold down a job, they cease to become eligible partners for marriage, and while they father children they evade a father's responsibility. In such neighbourhoods the middle class withdraws, social and economic isolation increases to constrain significantly the life chances of children and families who reside there (Wilson 1987).

Whereas Wilson was careful to analyse the *structural* causes of such behaviour, other commentators such as Charles Murray (1994) saw the picture the other way around and blamed the creation of an 'underclass' in deprived neighbourhoods, characterised by high rates of crime, family breakdown and welfare dependency. Such behaviour, he argued, rested on the poor moral choices of the residents that led to children born 'out of wedlock', fatherless families and delinquent youth. Thus an important debate was launched as to where the source and responsibility lay for urban disadvantage: from the habits and character of 'the poor' or the structure of inequality and segregation within the areas in which they lived.

This debate between what can be called 'structural' or 'constraint' theory of behaviour on one side and a moral and individual theory of personal irresponsibility on the other is critical for social workers to understand since it is precisely the *behavioural aspects* of disadvantage, poverty and social exclusion that they are dealing with on a day-to-day basis. It is important for social workers to reflect on the sources of behaviour represented in the debate between Wilson and Murray and the scores of commentators who have followed them. The 'going local' approach in this volume clearly sides with the general perspective that disadvantaged neighbourhoods drastically reduce the range of choices open to individuals and families with the inescapable corollary that the neighbourhood is a target for direct intervention. (For Wilson's important views on disadvantage and segregation in Britain see Wilson 1996.)

ACTIVITY 1.1: IDENTIFYING NEIGHBOURHOOD CHARACTERISTICS

Choose a neighbourhood as defined in this chapter that you are familiar with – where you work or live – and answer the following questions. What is the extent of mutual trust among neighbours? When school is in session would an adult be likely to ask a school-age child that they see out at the shops why he or she is not in school? Would adults intervene if they saw youths vandalising a tree? Bullying another child? Being cruel to an animal? Are there spaces beyond the control of public authorities? Is damage to public property left unrepaired (for example graffiti)?

But such a structural approach also acknowledges the complexity of the relationship between individuals and their local environments. It is not a question of simple determinism. Xavier de Souza Briggs argues that 'causal pathways' link residents' exposure to particular neighbourhood features to adverse social outcomes. For example, the behaviour of influential peer groups or parental networks in a neighbourhood can feed into patterns of anti-social behaviour and crime, school performance, and job finding for young people. Briggs provides another example of a causal pathway: crime and other stressors in the immediate environment can be linked to parenting efficacy and child development, and an adult's later mental health problems (Briggs 2004). Nevertheless the overall dynamic between families and the neighbourhoods and communities in which they live is subtle and complex. It is difficult to attribute causal effects to specific neighbourhood features and to know whether those effects are separable and additional to family characteristics or are mediated by or interactive with them. Sometimes only the broadest generalisations are possible: for example, 'neighbourhood crime is detrimental for residents' well being' or 'visible deterioration in the housing stock of a particular neighbourhood undermines quality of life'. As Briggs says, the key questions remain about these effects: 'how much, to whom, and with what longer-run effects . . .?' (Briggs 2004: 4).

ACTIVITY 1.2: HOW FAR CAN PRACTITIONERS TACKLE NEIGHBOURHOOD DISADVANTAGE?

Here is a thought experiment to see how much scope you might have in developing neighbourhood interventions. Consider the following scenarios:

1. *If* it could be shown that working individually with young people at risk of offending had no impact on youth crime in a particular area but that it was proven that a concerted, integrated effort by all youth agencies to increase job training in that area – by pooling budgets, bringing parents into close consultation, talking to employers, holding joint sessions with other service agencies – would you or your agency be willing to shift the focus of your work away from individual young people and towards community wide responses such as convening parent groups or meeting with other service practitioners?
2. Assume there is a shortage of foster parents in your locality and that earlier campaigns to recruit foster parents based on the needs of specific children have failed. You and your team have been approached by an alliance of voluntary organisations and community groups who aim to underscore the importance and the rewards of volunteering across the entire community. They intend to initiate a general campaign to recruit volunteers and are willing to include fostering under its umbrella. Would you be willing and able to contribute to that campaign? If not, why not? If so, what skills and perspectives would you bring to the consortium?

Research findings on neighbourhood effects

A formidable amount of neighbourhood-level research exists that examines the scale of effects on different aspects of family life and the individual life course. Major studies have collected much needed data linking the intensity of social problems and the behaviour of individuals with living in high-poverty neighbourhoods (Jargowsky 1996; Brooks-Gunn *et al.* 1997).

A number of impressive findings have followed up Wilson's path-breaking research and identified a range of effects after differences in individual characteristics have been controlled (Dietz 2002; Diez-Roux 2001). These show that neighbourhood conditions affect:

- local labour markets
- peer groups
- the social conduct of neighbours
- aspects of the physical or built environment

- the quality of services offered
- prevailing social norms
- levels of health and well-being
- quality of social interactions and networks
- the number and type of local institutions and organisations.

All of the above in turn shape the behaviour and life choices of local people. (For two excellent if detailed reviews of the literature of neighbourhood effects see Dietz 2002 and Sampson *et al*. 2002.)

Other studies have illuminated the range of such neighbourhood effects in specific ways:

- Child and adolescent outcomes such as infant mortality, low birth weight, teenage childbearing, school exclusion and drop-out rates, child abuse and neglect and anti-social behaviour by young people are all linked to neighbourhood (Brooks-Gunn and Aber 1997). Accidental injury, suicide of young people are also linked (Almgren in Sampson *et al*. 2002).
- Where ethnic minorities are concentrated in relatively deprived urban areas employment prospects are affected with, for example, higher rates of unemployment and lower rates of self-employment than ethnically balanced areas (Clark and Drinkwater 2002).
- There is a profound negative effect on pre-school children exposed to neighbourhood violence (Farver and Natera 2000).
- Neighbourhoods impact on a range of health outcomes, whether low birth weight, health protective behaviours, levels of adult mortality, cardiovascular risk factors and many others (Diez-Roux 2001; Morris *et al*. 1996; Acheson 1998; Browning and Cagney 2002).
- A link between the prevalence of crime within neighbourhoods and the 'efficacy' of neighbourhoods, that is the effectiveness within which social norms are projected and protected (Sampson *et al*. 2002).

BOX 1.2: NEIGHBOURHOODS: SPRINGBOARDS, TRAPS, OR STEPPING STONES?

Xavier de Souza Briggs (2004) proposes that neighbourhoods be roughly categorised as springboards, stepping stones or traps.

Traps: high-risk, low-resource neighbourhoods that tend to isolate families, meet few needs, and make it harder for families to move to better environments; they significantly compromise family well-being and may make it more difficult for families to see clearly the choices ahead of them, let alone pursue them – such as other housing elsewhere, better ways to manage their children (restrict contact with anti-social peer groups). In these contexts successful parenting requires a very high degree of buffering from neighbourhood risks and extreme resourcefulness in linking children or other family members to resources (since those resources are

continued

located elsewhere). Traps may be thought of as places that overwhelm the capacity to buffer risk of the typical family. When given some menu of exit options, most families who can leave will.

Stepping stones: offer moderate but important resources along with some risks, resources that help families hold ground but more often get ahead. These neighbourhoods meet key family needs, though successful parenting still requires active buffering from risks and active linking to resources. Families are able to gain resilience, though many will move out if conditions do not improve.

Springboards: low-risk, high-resource neighbourhoods that meet a range of family needs most of the time. They offer the most desirable set of resources all around. Few families will choose to move out without a radical shift in household composition or economic status (e.g. divorce, loss of job, needy relative requiring care).

THE DEMOCRATIC IMPERATIVE: GRASSROOTS MEET THE GRASSTOPS

A second driver pushing social work towards a more community-oriented practice is 'the democratic imperative'. There is a growing consensus that the degree of political control exercised by citizens at local level in Britain compares unfavourably to most European countries and others of the developed world (Jenkins 2004). This relative lack of local influence is not just a formal political question but has implications for the way services are provided. Personal public services, in particular, are now ripe for delivering at neighbourhood level. The compelling argument is emerging that responsibility for such services be 'transferred downwards to the lowest level at which it can effectively be discharged – the neighbourhood level' (John Smith Institute quoted in Jenkins 2004: 109). Jenkins cites the Scandinavian system, which places most personal services with the exception of health at the lowest identifiable tier of local government, no matter how small, including town and parish councils. The upshot is that for personal services 'contact between supplier and user is more effective because each in some degree knows the other' (Jenkins 2004: 108). This notion of the relational basis of service provision is key and should come naturally as it has long formed the cornerstone of social work and social care. It is found in other public services such as teaching and is also the foundation for the work faith institutions carry out in their communities.

The concept of 'strong democracy', in which citizens take on responsibility for governing themselves, provides a test and a marker for the future, not just in policy formation but in implementation. As one advocate writes 'A strong democracy should promote strong citizenship and a strong society. Giving people more and better opportunities to take part in their own governance can transform them from subjects of particular governmental arrangements to citizens vested in and supportive of those arrangements' (Thomas 1995: 7). 'Such citizens govern themselves directly . . . in particular when basic policies are being decided and when significant power is being deployed' (Barber 2003: 151). For years 'participation' and 'citizen involvement' have been conducted from the point of view of services themselves. Now mere compliance on the part of citizens is not sufficient because it is not effective. 'Whether learning new ideas or new skills, acquiring healthier habits, or changing one's outlook on family or society [only the people] can accomplish the change' (Thomas 1995: 7).

GOVERNMENT POLICY AND THE 'NEW LOCALISM'

The third driver pushing social work and social care towards more explicit and deeper involvement in neighbourhoods and communities is government policy, which, since 1997, has compelled public services to think local, to tailor services to local needs and to engage with local communities.

A number of policy initiatives have accelerated the urgency with which public services are to work more closely with and in localities. For example, neighbourhood renewal strategy urges services to join together to overcome the disadvantage and social exclusion of citizens living in the 88 most deprived areas of Britain (Cabinet Office 2000), while neighbourhood management is strongly advocated as a dominant paradigm for providing local services, not just in the original neighbourhood management pathfinders but across all urban areas (Power and Bergin 1999; PAT 4 2000).

The concept of neighbourhood management developed in the late 1990s out of a close analysis of what was actually happening in middle- and low-income urban areas. Groundbreaking research by Anne Power and colleagues had shown that when faced with major problems local people had no idea who to turn to (Power and Bergin 1999). Those problems as experienced by local people often appeared huge and insoluble, for example a rise in the number of poorly behaved children in the local primary school, youths setting fire to abandoned cars, a spate of thefts, lack of sufficient home care provision to allow seniors to remain in their home, areas given over to drug taking or resident locals with evident mental health problems.

Neighbourhood management aims to overcome the feelings of powerlessness of local citizens living in disadvantaged areas by building community capacity, making it easier for local organisations to get funding and involving community and voluntary service organisations in service delivery. The policy is being far more widely applied precisely in order to overcome this gap between what mainstream services deliver and the kinds of outcomes that local people want. It requires core public services to focus resources on disadvantaged neighbourhoods, build collaboration among services and extend community engagement. Neighbourhood management (PAT 4 2000) means:

- providing a person of authority that local people can turn to when things go wrong
- ensuring resident participation and providing leadership from the community itself
- providing local people with the tools to overcome identified problems and achieve desired outcomes across health, social care, child development, education and community safety
- developing a planned approach to tackling problems and achieving outcomes
- creating new service delivery mechanisms that integrate local services and focus on delivering what local people want.

CASE STUDY 1.1:   CHESTERTON'S PLAN FOR THE NEIGHBOURHOOD MANAGEMENT OF SERVICES

In the Chesterton area of Newcastle-under-Lyme in Staffordshire a strong effort is under way to integrate services at neighbourhood level. The aim is to effect a cultural change in the outlook of those very services in terms of how they regard the local area and local people. In particular it wants to encourage services to move away from an inward looking perspective and the prevailing attitude that they exist only for the very neediest. Historically, access to services has been made difficult through a process in which people are screened out by drawing a heavy line around those who are *not* deemed eligible for services and closing the door to them.

The neighbourhood plan for services is based on principles of accessibility, devolution and citizen engagement, bringing oversight of services down to the lowest practical level. What is interesting is the determination to get all services working with *all sections of the community*. There is for example an acknowledged problem of there not being enough for young people to do, so opportunities for young people – dance and music, off-road motor biking and better sports facilities – are in development. Equally acknowledged, however, is the perceived threat that groups of young people present to local residents so that youth services are responding to this as well. In resolving such conflicts consultation and engagement are recognised as critical to long-term success.

On young people's needs the plan has this to say:

> Young people have a culture of gathering in relatively large groups, and given the lack of buildings for them to use in the evening they are going to be the greatest users of public spaces after dark as places to socialise. As this group is also most likely to be the victims of violent crime, their needs have to be a priority. The intensification of lighting where paths cross or abut areas of public open space provide a greater sense of safety for all users, young and old.

What is striking in the plan is the strong visual element of the locality that comes through. Contributors from services and community have clearly mapped the neighbourhood in terms of need, and that sense of concrete street-level detail is evident. Environmental conditions and the signals they send to residents are prominently mentioned. Specific play areas, recreation grounds and sports facilities are identified, as are specific roads and the traffic hazards they present to residents. The work of community safety officers sits next to a paragraph on overgrown shrubbery (allowing cover for 'imagined assailants') and in turn moves onto alcohol abuse and domestic violence.

(Drawn from *Greater Chesterton Neighbourhood Action Planning Project*, 2006)

Government has developed its neighbourhood thinking in relation to specific services through a stream of green and white papers such as *Every Child Matters* (HM Treasury 2003), *Youth Matters* (DfES 2005b), and the white paper on social care *Our Health, Our Care, Our Say* (DoH 2006a). Collectively these specify higher levels of community engagement services for children and families, young people and adults. Across the board government is urging local services to draw local and community organisations into alliances and partnerships for service development and provision. It is asking services to develop high levels of participation and to give local citizens significant influence over defining need and shaping services to meet that need. In all dimensions of social care and social work, whether in assessment, planning and implementation and whether in services for older people, disabled people, adults and young people with a drug problem, family support and early years work, the imperative is there to increase participation, to build community capacity, to focus on the user's environment and above all to deliver on powerful outcomes to do with citizen well-being and a flourishing life.

Local authorities have responded to this agenda by creating locality teams, area implementation schemes, neighbourhood and consultative forums, decentralisation and one-stop shops in neighbourhoods, which are all indicative of the new localism. The new localism has also impacted on specific services in a number of ways: building services around institutions within those areas such as nurseries, schools, community centres and health centres.

Perhaps the most significant signal is that local authorities have also been thinking hard in terms of neighbourhoods as the point for service delivery. They are looking at their geographical area in terms of smaller, coherent localities, assembling data and mapping need more carefully in relation to neighbourhoods. Using vastly improved information systems they are developing databases useful for the public and practitioners alike in order to provide profiles on housing, poverty levels, health and social care data, faith and ethnicity, and educational attainment. These valuable data sets, which previously might have taken a community social work team months to assemble, are now readily available to practitioners in most cities and towns.

DEVELOPING COMMUNITY PRACTICE IN SOCIAL WORK AND SOCIAL CARE

Neighbourhood work and the social work role

There is widespread agreement that social work is committed to social justice and that it endeavours to assist, support and enable those who suffer from the effects of social exclusion and poverty. The International Association of Schools of Social Work and the International Federation of Social Work have defined the mission in the following way:

> The social work profession promotes social change, problem-solving in human relationships and the empowerment and liberation of people to enhance well-being. Utilising theories of human behaviour and social systems, social work intervenes at points where people interact with their environments. Principles of human rights, preserving human dignity and social justice are fundamental to social work.
>
> (IFSW 2000)

To put these principles into practice entails moving beyond the conventional frames of work with individuals and families to a fuller recognition of the interdependence between people and local environments, and a willingness to act as a change agent in those environments. Social work in its span of activities, roles and responsibilities is driven by a set of core values. While this is by no means a unique phenomenon (other professions and occupations hold values just as deeply) social work values orient its activities strongly in the direction of defending and expanding human rights and human dignity while tackling the inequities and injustices in society. Feminist practice, rural development projects and human rights advancement have all contributed to a range of interventions that step well outside the individual, psychologistic frames of reference of conventional casework practice.

In the US too, where privatised therapeutic and clinical models have dominated for so long, community practice is being explored with great urgency (Specht and Courtney 1994; Weil and Gamble 2005). Melvin Delgado has written persuasively about community capacity enhancement and the role of mapping the local geography as the means to change local environments. This assets perspective is based on five assumptions about the community in which the social worker functions: i) the community has the will and resources to help itself; ii) it knows what is best for itself; iii) ownership of the strategy rests within, rather than outside, the community; iv) partnerships involving organisations and communities are the preferred route for initiatives; v) using strength in one area will translate into strengths in other areas (Delgado 2000: 28).

Social work with individuals and families	Social work as community practice
Response to individual need, not social environment	Response to community need or problem collectively identified; (individual and family needs seen as aspect of common problems)
Relies on 'myth of intimacy' (of relationship between professional and client)	Community capacity enhancement – residents playing active and significant role
Underestimation of neighbourhood capacity while exaggerating weakness and needs	Acknowledges residents' difficulties in participation
Assessment (gathering information) of individual need	Asset-based assessment • Reflects local norms and experiences to minimise bias of practitioner • Local residents play an active and meaningful role throughout all phases (including being trained and hired) • Practitioners seek community input into programme design • Builds upon previous assessments/achievements
Any 'strengths based work' done with individuals and families only; does not extend to neighbourhoods	Strengths of community utilised; sees local environment as important target of intervention: schools, housing, social networks
Individual case planning	Service planning is a joint resource for whole neighbourhood and is outcome-focused

FIGURE 1.1 Key differences between social work focusing on individuals and families and social work geared for neighbourhood practice. (Adapted from Delgado 2000)

In the United Kingdom the Scottish Executive's report on social work in the twenty-first century, *Changing Lives*, is also very clear on the nature of the mission:

> Community social work has, in the past, been promoted as a discrete activity, conducted apart from mainstream social work practice. A new approach is now needed, which positions social work services at the heart of communities delivering a combination of individual and community based work alongside education, housing, health and police services.
>
> (Scottish Executive 2006)

The report foresees a needed strategic change of roles so that they:

- refocus on prevention and early intervention
- design and deliver services around the needs of individuals and communities, having local citizens participate in the design and purpose of the very services they receive
- manage knowledge explicitly by creating and maintaining learning networks that circulate concepts, data, information and solutions to highly complex social problems
- work collaboratively across public, voluntary and private sectors in tackling complex social problems that undermine citizen well-being in particular areas
- tackle social polarisation, inequality and social exclusion.

This enlarged mission means tackling some of the most persistent problems in British social life: the gap in life expectancy between social classes; families where no parents work; the link between low social and economic status and the likelihood of becoming addicted to drugs and alcohol; being either a victim or perpetrator of crime (Scottish Executive 2006; Jones *et al.* 2005).

Using social work skills in community practice

The means for working in and with neighbourhoods and communities grow organically out of current practice. As we will illustrate in the following chapters, many social work roles and responsibilities in specific service areas are already embracing a neighbourhood and community dimension. More than that, some of social work's longstanding assets can be brought directly into play. One such asset is practitioners' understanding of the life course and how that develops within a social and interactive framework. In his seminal paper Briggs ties the neighbourhood environment to a person's life course. He argues that it is not just the neighbourhood dynamics that have to be examined but how the individual came into that particular neighbourhood and what he or she does with their life once there (Briggs 2002: 26). Social workers are among the few human service practitioners who are trained and uniquely placed to understand this connection between individual and environment and to work with that relationship.

A second social work asset is its skill in building and maintaining relationships. Relationships, often through one-to-one encounters with residents, users and other professionals, is at the heart of neighbourhood work. Harnessing these relational skills for neighbourhood work is simply moving them to another stage.

A third asset is its understanding of power and how discriminatory or exclusionary power works to disadvantage users. In none of these areas do practitioners need 're-education', as a moment's reflection on comparison with health personnel will reveal.

BOX 1.3: A PROFESSION ALREADY IN TRANSITION? SOCIAL WORK POSTS WITH A COMMUNITY OR NEIGHBOURHOOD ORIENTATION

Social work and social care practice is already orienting itself more towards holistic community and neighbourhood intervention, with a proliferation of posts that place communities at least nominally as the target.

Project managers for engagement and participation with in Change for Children Programmes; children' centre staff providing a wide range of family support; care services for older people provided by adult and community services departments; Sure Starts for older people combining social care, education, health care and family support; supported housing and tenancy support which provides job finding and independent skills training; community drug projects; continuing care for people coming out of hospital.

KEY POINTS

☐ Neighbourhoods and geographical communities deeply affect the lives of the people who live in them. Research over the last dozen years into 'neighbourhood effects' has established that people's well-being and the kinds of social problems they have to wrestle with are shaped by the structure and dynamics of the neighbourhoods in which they live.

☐ Contemporary definitions of both 'neighbourhood' and 'community' accept that practitioners and policy makers cannot assume a common spirit of pulling together or a single viewpoint that represents 'community' opinion. Both concepts, however, refer to geographical areas that contain assets that social workers can use to improve outcomes for their users.

☐ Government policy is providing a strong impetus to localise services, engage communities and set up chains of influence so that local people have 'voice'. The neighbourhood management paradigm for services is now dominant.

☐ Social work is best seen as an ensemble of linked activities, spread across many diverse specialisms and occupations. Its tasks in the twenty-first century involve negotiating, brokering, networking, partnering and advocating. These relatively new tasks and approaches can only be carried out through a wider familiarity with the local neighbourhood environments and their impact on the lives of citizens.

☐   Social work already has a number of skill assets that can prove effective in community-based work. These are the capacity to link the wider environment to a person's life course, skills in relationship building, particularly active listening, a profound understanding of how power works and an historic commitment to combating oppression and working for social justice. Well-established skills that help people reach for the services right for them are also critical.

CHAPTER 2

UNDERSTANDING COMMUNITY PRACTICE

OBJECTIVES

By the end of this chapter you should:

- Be familiar with the difference between *community-level* services and *community-based* services

- Have a working definition of community practice

- Know some of the specific sources of information available on the neighbourhoods in which you work

- Be familiar with the four pillars of community practice: capacity building, outcomes, prevention, and knowledge management.

There are many different approaches to working with communities. Some, like community work or community organising, developed forty years ago or more. Others are blending older approaches with newer forms of community intervention. Often these newer approaches are based in specific services or are developing within services to specific groups of people, for example families with children under five, young people dependent on drugs, or older people who want to remain engaged in their neighbourhood. The concept of 'community practice' embraces this newer range of practitioners, who may be social workers, police officers, housing officers, community artists, youth workers or health workers, who have a community dimension to their work. Their roles and responsibilities require them to get to know their community's people and social circumstances, activate supporting networks, assist community groups to form and evolve, and develop links with community organisations. To do this they are developing new tools and approaches and hybrid roles. Although they remain practitioners based in public or voluntary organisations and continue to perform the tasks long associated with these organisations, they are also undertaking a range of community interventions.

THE DIFFERENCE BETWEEN 'COMMUNITY-LEVEL' AND 'COMMUNITY-BASED' SERVICES

When looking at the wide range of approaches and interventions for communities it is helpful to distinguish between those interventions that are *community-based* and those that are at *community level* (Barnes *et al.* 2006). Both provide services to people and both are geographically based but they work in different ways and with different objectives. Community-level interventions aim at the whole community and intend to change that community as their first priority and not necessarily to help specific families or people in need. This type of intervention, Barnes and her colleagues say, is based on the conviction 'that social problems, especially those created by disadvantage, are best dealt with by "capacity building" [in] the community rather than by identifying individuals with problems and providing services to them' (Barnes *et al.* 2006: 87). The aim is to improve levels of well-being across the whole community for all who live there. The assumption behind community-level intervention is that a vigorous community that has the capacity to solve problems will be able to provide a high level of well-being for those who live there. In short it seeks to change the community rather than individuals.

Community-based interventions seek to do the opposite. They aim to meet the needs of individuals and families through services and supports in the community. Services are typically available through common access points, such as local schools or health clinics, local offices or through drop-in centres and outreach work. Referrals tend to be self-initiated and informally dealt with. The outcome of this kind of intervention is to accomplish change in levels of well-being for individuals and families, while any capacity building for the community as a whole is a by-product of the service.

Many programmes do both and strive to add to a community's capacity and improve levels of well-being and at the same time offer services and support to individuals and families. Indeed, there is a close connection between the two (Barnes *et al.* 2006). Sure Start Children's Centres, discussed at greater length in Chapter 5, provide a good example. Their objective is to raise the standards of parenting and child development across the whole of the neighbourhoods in which they are situated. But they also provide services to individual families, for example providing child care, speech therapy or support for mothers with post-natal depression. In practice it is often difficult to pinpoint where the community-based service ends and the community-level activities begin.

DEFINING COMMUNITY PRACTICE

The number of jobs in the voluntary and public sector with a community dimension is proliferating. All major services are developing a 'community' side to them, whether policing, social work and social care, housing, health or education. Much of this has happened informally without a strong blueprint to follow. This makes any attempt to define this breadth of activity in a single phrase very difficult. In general 'community practice' is now widely used as an umbrella for the range of tasks, roles and responsibilities that are emerging from many different sources. Banks defines community practice as including 'all of those processes that are about stimulating, engaging and achieving 'active community' (Banks *et al.* 2003: 15).

BOX 2.1: COMMUNITY PRACTICE

Community practice refers to work which takes place on three different levels. These correspond to the levels of intervention outlined in ecological theory and as such should be familiar to social workers. These are:

- practice at community or neighbourhood level with a focus on 'micro-level' activities – including capacity building, community development and community education;
- practice at organisational/inter-organisational level such as service development and outreach, community liaison, partnership formation, community service provision;
- practice at societal level including activities to modify institutions, shape cultural debates and intervene in politics and debates about social justice and citizenship.

The purposes of community practice include the following:

- improving quality of life;
- extending human rights and deepening democracy, particularly by participatory structures;
- advocacy for communities of interest such as children with behavioural problems;
- community capacity building which assists localities in developing the skills and resources to control more of their own services and public life;
- service integration and provision of new services;
- social justice.

The practitioner aiming to provide services that address the well-being of an entire neighbourhood or geographical community takes on certain additional responsibilities in relation to their service role. They are:

- to undertake participative service planning on the basis of assessment of community concerns;
- to consult and negotiate with stakeholders, local people and other participants in the neighbourhood;
- to foster collaborative approaches committed to inter-agency and holistic services;
- to work within an environment of diversity, fluidity and often conflict;
- to develop participative approaches to enhance neighbourhood resources and commitment to organisational learning;
- to promote local leadership.

(Adapted from Banks *et al.* 2003)

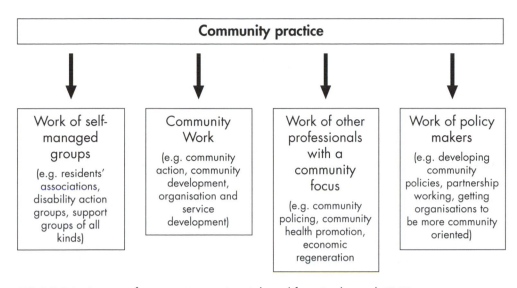

FIGURE 2.1 Aspects of community practice. Adapted from Banks *et al.* 2003

ACTIVITY 2.1: SITUATING SERVICE AGENCIES IN NEIGHBOURHOOD AND COMMUNITY

On the following page is a scatter plot with two axes. The axis running from top to bottom represents different sizes of geographical areas – with the largest area (region) at the top and the smallest (a street) at the bottom. The axis that bisects it runs from left to right, with highest input of professional expertise at the left and the highest input of local citizen knowledge on the right. Think of an area you work in and then locate the organisations listed in the boxed column to the right at different points on the plot as you would find them in your area. It is important to do this in relation to a neighbourhood you are familiar with since the position of the organisations may well be different in different areas. If the services listed in the box are not found in your neighbourhood think of others and situate them instead. Several organisations have already been plotted as examples.

There are four pillars of enduring importance to community practice. First is the commitment to building the skills, abilities and motivation of local people and local organisations to tackle the 'wicked' issues which beset their own neighbourhood and community. This is often broadly referred to as *capacity building*, in the sense of developing competences in depth not just to solve local problems but to fashion an environment after their own wishes. Second is *outcomes*, those universal attainments for human flourishing that all people want for themselves and their families. Third is the commitment to *prevention*, a practice that moves 'upstream' in order to tackle the sources of social problems before they emerge. Fourth is *knowledge management* – gathering data, information and local knowledge and organising it for effective action.

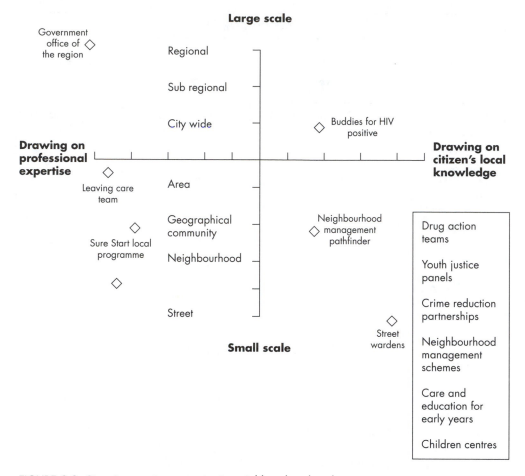

Large scale

Regional

Sub regional

City wide

Drawing on professional expertise

Area

Geographical community

Neighbourhood

Street

Small scale

Government office of the region

Leaving care team

Sure Start local programme

Drawing on citizen's local knowledge

Buddies for HIV positive

Neighbourhood management pathfinder

Street wardens

Drug action teams

Youth justice panels

Crime reduction partnerships

Neighbourhood management schemes

Care and education for early years

Children centres

FIGURE 2.2 Situating service agencies in neighbourhood and community

COMMUNITY CAPACITY BUILDING

While public services help create benefits for local people they cannot do so on their own. Health services for children or older people, maintaining community safety, educational attainment and reducing anti-social behaviour are all, to one degree or another, reliant on the capacities and strengths of the neighbourhoods in which those services are delivered. Families have an important role in ensuring the health and educational progress of their children. Community safety is maintained not just by policing, but in the willingness of the community to visibly and publicly uphold certain norms of behaviour. Older people remain in their own homes not only because of the strength of the local health and social care systems but also because informal social supports are available. The capacity of neighbourhoods to contribute in this way is critical to the success or failure of public services.

When we refer to 'capacity' in relation to communities and neighbourhoods we mean their ability to act in particular ways, with specific faculties or powers to do or accomplish tasks (Chaskin *et al.* 2001). Having capacity enables localities to recognise common problems and set in train the arrangement of resources and assets it needs to deal with these problems.

BOX 2.2:   COMMUNITY CAPACITY BUILDING: A DEFINITION

Chaskin and his colleagues define capacity building this way:

Community capacity is the interaction of human capital, organisational resources and social capital existing within a given community that can be leveraged to solve collective problems and improve or maintain the well-being of that community. It may operate through informal social processes and/or organised efforts by individuals, organisations, and social networks that exist among them and between them and the larger systems of which the community is a part.

(Chaskin *et al.* 2001: 7)

Capacity building contributes to the growth of assets such as 'human capital', which includes the skills, knowledge and abilities of those who live in the area. It also builds 'social capital', which includes the social networks, the sense of trust and the willingness to volunteer. It does not mean leaving a community to solve its own problems, but it does mean assisting local people and local organisations to acquire skills and knowledge that will allow them to direct or influence the response to problems they identify. This can take place at different levels and in different directions. Augmenting the influence of local people over issues that concern them, improving the skills of local people to address public and private issues, and improving and focusing collective energies to address particular problems: this is what capacity building means.

Briggs' (1997) key observation that advocacy and place are interlinked is a unifying thread bringing together approaches that link work with individuals and families with that of neighbourhoods and communities. For example, capacity building can mean putting in place the conditions in which local residents gain some experience of wielding influence and power – developing leaders, learning to deal with the media, running meetings, giving voice to community aspirations. In this sense it means equipping residents to 'gain a seat at the table' and to contribute in an informed, potent way to public discussions where important decisions are taken that affect that neighbourhood.

It can also include raising the level of volunteering in the neighbourhood, bringing together peer mentors for younger pupils at risk of school exclusion, creating litter patrols, starting up a youth centre, convening a young persons' parish council, setting up informal neighbourhood care schemes or starting a consultation exercise over a neighbourhood ten-year plan.

Local communities have, of course, different levels of resources that people can draw on – whether the quality of services such as schools or health clinics, their housing and physical infrastructure or their connection to the jobs market and levels of income. Often these resources are distributed – and segregated – unequally along lines of race, ethnicity, social class and gender. Given this overall pattern of inequality and of huge differences in resources it is still feasible to talk about community capacity in a general sense.

BOX 2.3: EIGHT DOMAINS OF COMMUNITY CAPACITY

Laverack and Labonte, working in Canada, have laid out eight domains to planning a community framework for health promotion that are equally useful for social care provision and children and family outcomes (Laverack and Labonte 2000). The eight domains are:

Participation

Only by participating in small groups, forums, user groups or larger organisations can individuals add their voice to definitions of concerns and proposed solutions; equally, unless citizens collectively have a 'seat at the table' and channels of influence open to them neighbourhood concerns and propositions will not be heard by service providers.

Leadership

Participation and leadership are interconnected; leadership needs to be nurtured and mentored and requires a strong participant base to produce it, just as participation requires the direction and structure of strong leadership. Both participation and leadership play an important role in the development of community groups and neighbourhoods finding their 'voice'.

Organisational/institutional structures

These include committees, associations, clubs, faith institutions and youth groups. They represent both the ways and the means by which people come together in small institutions in which they have influence in order to socialise and address concerns and problems; the range and capacity of such organisations together with the networks they spawn are critical to a community's capacity.

Problem assessment

The capacity to identify problems and concerns, together with proposed solutions and actions to resolve them, are central to a community's ability to be an effective partner.

Resource mobilisation

The ability of the community to mobilise resources from within and to negotiate resources from beyond itself is an important factor in its capacity to resolve problems it faces.

'Asking why'

The ability to critically assess the social, political and economic cause of inequalities and sources of disadvantage is an important step in assembling public strategies.

Links with others

This is the ability to form alliances, partnerships and collaborations and to use independent experts, researchers and intermediaries who may be able to amass critical resources like knowledge or funding. It also includes access to formal and informal resources, inter-organisational networks, creating a sense of collective action and shared core values. While it is relatively easy to create and maintain links within particular services, it is more difficult to undertake this work in relation to other agencies and groups engaged in broad-based capacity building and other advocacy-oriented organisations.

Community control over programme

This takes time and resources; as programmes become more complex and demanding of those resources, it becomes more difficult for local people to maintain influence within service programmes. Yet that is the very purpose of community capacity building.

Approaches to capacity building

Health care services in Europe, Canada, the US and to a lesser extent the UK have realised that community capacity building strategies can lead to innovative practice. They have already begun to implement community-based interventions that combine education around risk factors with medical treatment for those most at risk using a broad mix of behavioural, social-change and community-development models (Mittelmark 1999: 7). What all such community development models have in common is a process that, according to Mittelmark (1999: 19):

- emphasises the participation of people in their own development (as opposed to the 'client state')
- recognises and uses people's assets (as opposed to attending mainly to their problems and limitations)
- encourages the participation of people in the generation of information about community needs and assets (as opposed to research controlled by professionals)
- empowers people to make choices (as opposed to the management of people by institutions of power)
- involves people in the political processes that affect their lives (as opposed to nonparticipation).

The Acheson Report (1998) on the relation between health inequalities and geography influenced health professionals in shifting their attention from a concentration on the individual to a focus on the individual as part of a neighbourhood environment. The government white paper *Our Healthier Nation* (DoH 1998) also explicitly recognised the importance of the links between health and local social problems. Health Action Zones embraced essentially a capacity building approach and achieved a great deal in a short time in tackling health inequalities locally (Maddock, 2000).

Social work is also beginning to realise that it, along with all other major service providers, has a role to play in community capacity building. Delgado in the US, for example, stresses the need to focus on neighbourhood assets, to learn from them, draw on them, develop them and build them. 'The adoption of a deficit perspective has diverted much time and energy from the development of an asset perspective; in essence the process of "retooling" that is necessary has suffered from misguided foci' (Delgado 2000: 25–26).

Social work's contribution to building community capacity can only be made in collaboration with other services and local people. While health or education services can initiate their own self-standing capacity building programmes around, for example, a 'healthy community' or a 'community that learns', social work, because of its intermediary position, cannot do this. That does not mean, however, that it has no contribution to make to community capacity building. On the contrary, its perceptions of power and empowerment and its long-standing commitment to tackle racism, oppression and social injury make it an effective catalyst. While succeeding chapters in this volume explain this capacity building role in relation to particular services and projects, it is worth reflecting on the approaches to power and relationships that social work can bring to capacity building in communities and neighbourhoods.

CASE STUDY 2.1: CAPACITY BUILDING IN NORWICH

For many years Norwich had a history of community development work focusing mainly on pulling together residents' associations and finding, utilising and maintaining community meeting venues. But there was a missing dimension – the democracy dimension – and the local authority wanted to explore the implication of community power more fully. A joint-services 'Democracy' working party was set up, bringing together senior officers from the local authority, health and police services, which then decided to set up a number of community forums.

Six community workers were given briefs to facilitate the development of community power by moving away from the historical emphasis on buildings. They called a series of area meetings at which they proposed to set up twelve area forums covering all wards in the city. Significantly, they did not set the boundaries but left it to residents to decide these according to their perceptions of neighbourhood. Once areas were defined there were elected representatives from each area who then constituted as a group within the city council.

The project learned by doing and quickly found out what it did not know. It was apparent that health services and police were wanting to formalise consultative channels for their own organisational purposes. The locally elected representatives were given training and encouraged to adopt a parish council model for consolidating their position. The representatives rejected that model, however, because of its lack of democracy – the continuous holding of office by a few. They opted instead for a direct democracy model. The representatives aimed to give local people the information on the scope of what they could decide. In effect they said, 'This is the picture, here's the area of flexibility in the budget where your decision will count, here are our present commitments.' In short they referred decisions on services back to their people, all the more impressive given that the project occurred within a context of public expenditure cuts from £26m down to £16m.

(Adapted from Reynolds 2006)

DELIVERING OUTCOMES

Outcomes are those broad and positive conditions that we all seek in order to enhance our well-being. Their significance for social work and social care cannot be exaggerated. Government has made specific outcomes imperative for all services, especially in relation to children, young people and older people as well as for neighbourhoods as a whole. Staying healthy, achieving specific goals, keeping secure and safe, and living in stimulating surroundings are all typical outcomes, the sorts of things that people desire for themselves. The outcome revolution in fact opens the door to a fuller conception of what social work should be striving for, namely to help secure the basis for human flourishing in concert with other services.

The very nature of outcomes imposes a powerful discipline on public services. To see why this is so we have to understand the essential difference between outcomes and other terms from new public management such as 'targets' or 'performance indicators'. There is for example a profound difference between outcome and output. Outputs are under the control of services themselves; they are essentially units of services offered or provided to users, whether places in an early years care and education nursery, the number of intermediate care plans offered older people or tenancies in supported housing units. Definitions of service success are much easier for service providers to describe in terms of outputs because they say nothing about the results and impact on people themselves. Did lives improve? Was there greater mobility, educational opportunity, higher levels of well-being? Such questions essentially lie outside the capacity of outputs to tell us.

Outcomes, on the other hand, are universal aims to be achieved within a particular service field towards which any particular set of service outputs or practitioner activity *may or may not* assist. The concept of outcome switches the focus away from the provider's perspective towards society-wide concepts of well-being for all citizens. Working towards outcomes should engender a sense of limits, even humility in practitioners – no one service could possibly think of achieving outcomes on its own. Rather they can only be achieved through collaboration.

Outcomes express universal conditions which *all* people, user and citizen alike, should enjoy. In this sense they are closely related to the concept of 'capabilities' developed by the United Nations Development Programme (UNDP), which are the minimum capacities that all people must have, wherever they live, in order to achieve a sense of well-being (UNDP 1995). Social work is not accustomed to thinking of its practice in this way, however. As such it is tempting for practitioners and their managers to dismiss any concerted effort to achieve outcomes because of certain practical difficulties, not least because service objectives are often about preventing harm and have a far shorter time frame.

The outcome revolution means, however, that decisions, whether strategic or operational, should be judged in terms of their impact on outcomes. In making decisions around eligibility or rationing services it is common to think of these as stand-alone alternatives (and often with a bias that presumes lack of eligibility). Take for example a decision on whether home care hours should be cut or the opening times reduced for a low-cost day centre for older people. While it looks as if this requires a decision on a straightforward trade-off between two types of resources for older people, both alternatives should first be looked at in terms of a projected impact on outcomes before the consequences of such a decision can be fully understood (Bardach 2005: 51). Which decision will contribute to better health or greater inclusion in the neighbourhood (or conversely do the least damage)? The outcomes for specific service areas are discussed more fully in Chapters 5 to 7.

PREVENTIVE WORK

'Preventive work' is intimately linked to a focus on outcomes. The phrase is something of a misnomer – after all *what* is actually being prevented? It takes on greater clarity when defined by its opposites such as 'reactive work' or 'crisis intervention'. Health promotion projects reveal clearly what is at stake in preventive work. One well-known example is in the field of cardiac services, where between 1997 and 2002 there was a decline of 23 per cent in deaths from heart disease. Some of this was a result of improved cardiac services, whether surgery or cholesterol-reducing drugs. But a good percentage was also because of improved life choices, whether diet, taking exercise or giving up smoking (Leadbetter 2004). This same double-pronged approach stressing both cure and prevention to a major health issue is found elsewhere: in young people and sexual health, or in understanding the importance of diet and healthy living during pregnancy. Social care and social work services have comparable arenas for preventive work. For example, in order to forestall social exclusion arising from low educational achievement social workers should be promoting stimulating environments for child development. Providing and promoting activities for young people in order to prevent or diminish anti-social behaviour in a particular locality is another example. Strengthening caring networks in a locality to reduce rates of older people going into hospital is a third. Yet the commitment to prevention has been taken on very slowly. Social work and social care have found it difficult to move beyond programmed responses to individual casualties of a winner/ loser society, almost inviting the perception that it is a residual service, the ultimate safety net.

The important element in preventive work, as Leadbetter notes,

> is a different account of the way public well-being is understood. With pre-ventive work as the dominant model the state does not act upon society, nor provide a curative or repair service. Instead the state creates a platform or an environment in which people take decisions about their lives in a different way. This is bottom-up, mass social innovation, enabled by the state.
>
> (Leadbetter 2004: 16)

Such a model does not inhibit effective top-down services provided by central or local government. Indeed, the capacity of government to provide more effective services directly to users may well depend on its capacity to encourage people to become more skilful in assessing and managing their own health, welfare and social needs (Leadbetter 2004).

Leadbetter argues that many of our biggest social challenges – reducing obesity and smoking, caring for people with chronic health conditions, promoting learning and creating safer communities – must rely on self-organising (i.e. by local citizens) solutions. 'Public service professionals', he writes, 'would help to create platforms and environments, peer-to-peer support networks, which allow people to devise these solutions collaboratively' (Leadbetter 2004: 16).

BOX 2.4: 'THE CHURCH OF ACCIDENTS': A PARABLE ABOUT PREVENTION

Once there was a church on a sharp bend of the road. It was built at the spot which the church founding fathers thought ideal in the years before the motor car when the only traffic that travelled along the road was carts and wagons. The first cars that came along were few in number and presented no hazard. But as the years went by the cars became bigger and faster. One day a driver failed to take the bend and crashed into a tree. He was hauled out with a broken leg. The very next week two more drivers suffered injuries in the same manner.

The congregation held a meeting to decide what to do. After much debate they set up a small volunteer rescue team with rudimentary first aid equipment available. It wasn't long before the team had a chance to show what it could do. One Sunday during service the congregation heard the high whine of a really powerful engine; they knew instinctively that the driver had no idea of the bend ahead. A few moments later there was an enormous crash outside. The team rushed out to offer what help they could but it was not enough. The driver was killed and members of his family in the car were distraught beyond consolation. The survivors were helped inside the church and comforted. 'I guess we'd better prepare ourselves for worse to come,' one parishioner said. And so the rescue team grew in size. It acquired sophisticated first aid equipment and established something further: a team of comforters and counsellors to help survivors recover from trauma and loss.

A great deal of information on different vehicles' safety records and causes of accidents was also amassed, while expertise steadily developed around responding to bereavement and offering appropriate help. Over time this became as much a focus of activity as worship and a great proportion of the church's budget was taken up funding this activity. 'We are nearly out of money,' the church elders said, 'what are we going to do?' Someone suggested, and it was agreed, that a charge be levied for the crash services that the church offered.

Things continued like this for another six months, until one Sunday when, after a particularly traumatic week, some of the church elders brought in a proposal that the accident and trauma team remain in place full time regardless of cost. At this point a young girl stood up in the congregation and said, 'But why don't we straighten out the bend in the road?' A stunned silence followed. Finally one elder said, 'But we can't do that. We don't have the expertise. We'd

continued

have to find others to help us and they would want to take over.' Another said, 'What would happen to our services? We have excellent services – we have helped hundreds of people to survive both physically and psychologically.' Another said, 'And what would our counsellors and first aid staff do – where would they go? What would happen to their expertise?' 'And don't forget our income, people,' said another. 'I don't want to sound materialistic but our services now do command fees that keep this place going.'

So the bend was not straightened out. And the accidents kept on happening.

LOCAL KNOWLEDGE

There has been a quantum leap since the year 2000 in the amount of concrete data now available to practitioners concerning the area in which they work. One of the initiatives to come out of the Strategy for Neighbourhood Renewal (Neighbourhood Renewal Unit (NRU) 2001) is the provision of neighbourhood and 'small area' data to a range of practitioners and the need for government to make this widely available through the National Statistics website (Policy Action Team 18 2000).

Neighbourhood statistics include census information and a breakdown of what the different indices of multiple deprivation indicate neighbourhood by neighbourhood. These indices, commissioned by the Neighbourhood Renewal Unit in 2004 from the Social Disadvantage Research Centre at Oxford University, combine separate domains of deprivation:

- income deprivation
- employment deprivation
- health deprivation and disability
- education, skills and training deprivation
- barriers to housing and services
- crime
- living environment deprivation.

In addition to these seven there are two other indices: income deprivation affecting children and income deprivation affecting older people (Office of the Deputy Prime Minister (ODPM) 2004).

Street-level data

Getting data specific to a practitioner's neighbourhood may depend on the kind of information wanted and how the neighbourhood's boundaries have been determined. The greatest amount of official data is usually available ward by ward but the neighbourhood of operation may not fit existing ward boundaries. If this is the case, it should be possible to take an average of the wards that are in and around the neighbourhood of concern, which would at least provide an approximation of data.

Highly local data, focused on only a few streets, is also available. These so-called 'super output areas' (SOAs) bring together a high volume of information provided for small target areas, so small that there may be several SOAs within a political ward. It may be possible to define your neighbourhood or district precisely by adding together several output areas. SOA data provides multiple data sets on key areas of neighbourhood life, which includes numbers of households with limiting long-term illness and dependent children, number of lone-parent households with dependent children, breakdown of ethnicity, economic activity and gender. More specifically SOA data includes:

- health and care data on life expectancy, hospital episodes, healthy lifestyle behaviours and provision of unpaid care
- crime and community safety data on crime, fires and road accidents
- community well-being information on community involvement, social inclusion and improving overall standards (e.g. street cleanliness)
- housing data sets on tenure and condition, overcrowding and homelessness
- economic deprivation data relating to economic activity, poverty and the provision of welfare benefits.

To access this information from the Office of National Statistics website practitioners need only a postcode or the name of an area they wish to explore. Other data sources are also highly relevant to filling out practitioner's understanding of the local social ecology. For example, the Department for Education and Skills (www. dfes.gov.uk) or the local authority can provide data on educational attainment at key stage 2, key stage 3, GCSE and A level results.

ACTIVITY 2.2: USING THE NATIONAL STATISTICS DATABASE

Go to the website of the Office of National Statistics (www.statistics.gov.uk) click on 'Neighbourhoods' and then enter in the search window a postcode or the name of a locality for which you are interested in collecting data.

While such statistics undoubtedly help central government decide where to target new initiatives they also give practitioners and local citizens a valuable tool in assessing conditions in local areas, deciding where to target their own resources locally and helping to keep track year on year in progress towards service outcomes by providing baseline figures to work against. Crime reduction programmes, services for older people, drug action teams, healthy schools and Sure Start children's centres were among the early cluster of local service initiatives to use such statistics. But their use extends in virtually every direction, and teams with even partial community orientation (such as children's safety or domestic abuse teams) need to take advantage of this. Most local authorities have established knowledge management units who will help practitioners assemble the data they need, but there is no substitute for exploring the web-based information for oneself.

Mapping

In organising and managing data and local knowledge it is important to think graphically using maps and other visual arrangements of data and information. Mapping is the general term for a range of depictions of resources, needs, assets and problems of a given neighbourhood. Mapping provides practitioners with a resource that can integrate large amounts of data. It can also be used to enhance capacity, since the process should involve local people, while graphic representation can be an immensely powerful tool in creating the kinds of collaboration we discuss below and provide ready material for public displays, public discussions and interaction with local residents.

The aims of any mapping process should be:

- to produce new insights about the neighbourhood that will lead to changes
- draw on widespread involvement of local people
- give direction for how to maximise local resources
- provide transferable skills for those who take part (Delgado 2000).

While social work has long mapped out social and familial relationships in devices such as eco maps this takes the process to a neighbourhood level. Drawing on the experiences of a neighbourhood in Los Angeles, Delgado notes that community mapping should consist of six steps: i) a clear definition of the area to be mapped; ii) the development of a process for formulating key questions that need to be answered during the mapping process; iii) the development of standardised methods for recording and portraying information, for example photographs, videotapes, audiotapes, diagrams; iv) the mapping process itself; v) analysis of information assembled and vi) presentation of results (Delgado 2000).

The value of hard data cannot be exaggerated. In forming the kinds of alliances and collaboratives discussed throughout this volume, one of the most powerful negotiating tools is hard new evidence or precise information which will buttress support for particular initiatives, and information and knowledge that will persuade would-be partners.

Such data sets need to be supplemented by drawing on local knowledge. Data sets only take practitioners so far; they are snapshots after all and the scene that they depict is ever changing. Involving local people in the gathering and systematising of information brings greater depth to understanding local data. Training local people in the use of surveys and questionnaires should also be provided. But just as importantly the continuity of local knowledge reaches dimensions that data sets cannot reach – the historical dimension, the movement and the changes in the locality over time.

BOX 2.5: NEIGHBOURHOOD AREA PROFILE: BURSLEM/COBRIDGE IN STOKE-ON-TRENT

The Knowledge Management Unit for Stoke-on-Trent has divided Stoke into 48 neighbourhoods. For one of these – Burslem and Cobridge – they provide the following profile*:

- *Population, faith and ethnicity*
  70 per cent of the population describes itself as white and 18 per cent as Pakistani. 54 per cent described their religion as Christian, 24 per cent as Muslim, and 21 per cent as having no religion.
- *Health and social care*
  23 per cent of the population between 16 and 64 had a limiting long-term illness, 17 per cent described their health as 'not good', 10 per cent provided unpaid care; life expectancy was six and a half years *less* than the national average ('years of life lost'), while the social services department had 63 users per 1000 compared with 46 per 1000 in the city at large.
- *Education*
  46 per cent of all pupils were eligible for free school meals (compared to 26 per cent across the city), 53 per cent of pupils have English as a second language, and educational attainment was significantly lower at all key stages compared to pupils across the city.
- *Housing*
  51 per cent were owner occupiers while 31 per cent rented from the council or a housing association; 10 per cent of all households were classified as overcrowded (twice the city average) while 15 per cent of households were without central heating.

*this is highly condensed from the data the Knowledge Management Unit holds on this particular neighbourhood. My thanks to Steve Johnston of the KMU for this information.

BOX 2.6: A BASIC WAY OF ORGANISING INFORMATION AT NEIGHBOURHOOD LEVEL

- *Headline indicators* or 'change indicators' measure important aspects of the neighbourhood (e.g. crime levels) and how they change over time. These are particularly useful for measuring progress towards outcomes.
- *Context indicators* provide background and descriptive information (either from neighbourhood statistics or one-off surveys). These might show the degree of economic deprivation or changes in ethnic make-up.
- *Service performance indicators* show how mainstream public services perform locally and are available from the Audit Commission (www.audit-commission.co.uk), which gathers data on the service performance indicators for local authorities, health trusts and the police.
  (NRU 2005)

CASE STUDY 2.2: COMMUNITY PRACTICE

On a moderate-sized housing estate on the edge of a large industrial city in the West Midlands the high levels of young people using drugs in a neighbourhood has a widespread impact. Many dimensions of neighbourhood life are affected:

- drug dealing is carried on before and after school just beyond the school perimeter
- drug-related litter is found on the small recreation ground
- a far corner of the neighbourhood, where boarded-up houses are situated, is used as a place to meet and deal
- a small number of house burglaries are committed by those who need to find ready cash to spend on their dependency.

A number of services are affected directly by this problem. Police have rising (but still modest) levels of crime to deal with, the secondary school is concerned that its reputation will falter, as the main housing provider the housing association is concerned that it is losing authoritative oversight of its property, and environmental services have increased amounts of litter to deal with – some of which is drug related. Residents feel that the sense of trust and of informal community controls that governed behaviour until recently have plummeted. Residents say they feel there is little they can do.

A social worker on the child and adolescent mental health services (CAMHS) team receives a referral for a 15-year-old male whose behaviour has led to his suspension from school. At home he stays in his room, where from time to time his parents have found drug paraphernalia. His one out-patient appointment with a child psychiatrist has suggested the possibility of a 'dual diagnosis', a reference to inter-related drug and mental health problems.

Clearly the worker will focus first on the needs of the family and of the 15-year-old with a developing drug dependency. But to do this the worker also needs to address, in collaboration with others, neighbourhood-level issues as well. The case work and neighbourhood work are intertwined; the young person's behaviour is enmeshed in neighbourhood behaviours possibly at a tipping point. It is arbitrary and counterproductive for the worker simply to draw a line around the young person and his family and say, 'that which is inside the circle is my business and that which is outside the circle is none of my business.'

Mapping provision

The social worker and her or his team may have already mapped out what services or resources are available in the area that relate to drug problems and young people. Any combination of these may prove helpful: a drop-in confidential advice service; residential beds in a nearby treatment clinic; a needle exchange; GPs who prescribe methadone; outreach youth workers; parent support or peer support groups; anti-bullying programmes at the secondary school; a community rehab programme.

Other neighbourhood-level links also become critical, and they too have questions to answer and resources to find.

Policing

What action are the police taking to tackle drug-related problems? Have they focused on the street dealing around the school? Are there street wardens or CCTV cameras that could be deployed to limit drug supply chains, particularly in the further corner of the estate? Are there locally targeted campaigns to encourage young people to 'say no' and/or to supply information about dealers in the vicinity?

Schools and youth service

Does the high school have a drugs policy? Does it run information and awareness nights for parents and their sons and daughters? Are there sexual health promotion clinics run off campus but publicised in school? Does the youth service provide programmes that address drug issues with young people or seek to engage young people through community arts or sports or detached youth-work programmes?

Public space and property

This is key since the use of public space is critical to how a neighbourhood understands itself and whether it believes it has the 'capacity' to deal with problems it feels strongly about. The 'broken windows' theory first advanced by Kelling and Wilson (1982) points to the consequences of allowing minor acts of vandalism and criminal damage, whether graffiti or indeed broken windows, to remain unrepaired. To do so gives a highly public signal that the area is not being looked after by either public authority or informal community authority and is therefore ripe for using for more serious criminal purposes. 'Fixing broken windows' is sometimes the more effective response to reducing criminal activity than 'incident oriented' policing.

In this scenario drug-related litter needs to be cleaned up with collection responsibilities pinpointed and public education campaigns instituted. The housing association should have an agreed policy on allocation of properties to drug users with local schemes to prevent tenancy breakdown and to manage anti-social behaviour related to drugs in the area.

The social work roles and responsibilities in this scenario will potentially be distributed across several teams and agencies: the drug action team, youth offending team, a school-based social worker, primary care trust based social worker, children and adolescent mental health team, specialist adolescent support team, family support team, youth projects run by voluntary organisation. Each of these in some way may be involved in both work with the family *and* in neighbourhood-level intervention.

The perspectives in the above study can be applied to different kinds of problems where individual behaviour is enmeshed with wider neighbourhood conditions. We can see the elements of capacity building that should interest social work, because they directly impact on the effectiveness with which social work can deliver outcomes. Investing in community capacity building is as important for social work as for any of the major services. Without such investment the means for achieving the outcomes for children, young people and older people will be severely constrained.

The principles of community practice suggest the following:

- Listen to local people define the problem. They will have a clear view of what is wrong ('parents who don't care', 'young people out of control', 'I can't go out on the streets at night') with firm views about how to set it right. But service providers may think they know what is best, may be reliant on 'silo' thinking with a very standard, limited capacity to respond to the specific problem, or claim they do not have the resources to tackle the problem at source. Listening to local people means using local networks, building relational empowerment and identifying 'communities of interest' within the locality.

- Measure the problem by finding out how big it is and how many people are actually affected, mapping as precisely as possible where and when the drug-related activities take place (dealing, burglary, littering, smoking) to get as accurate a view of the scale of the problem as possible. It is easy to understand how drug taking can mushroom as a source of apprehension and fear within a locality.

- Develop holistic thinking around responses: what particular courses of action or combined courses of action will retard, slow down or diminish the problem? Again, agencies need the views and assistance of local people. Silo thinking would have the various agencies proposing what they consider to be their ready, off-the-shelf responses to pre-selected problems. What is needed is some thinking around *why* the drug activity is happening and *why* particular sets of responses would work. This is developing a 'theory of change' – a theory as to why particular actions will produce improvement.

KEY POINTS

☐   Community practice is a fast-expanding area of service provision, embracing a wide range of practitioners drawn from the public and voluntary sectors who have some dimension of community or neighbourhood work in their roles and responsibilities. They include teachers and police officers, mental health workers, youth workers and social workers to name a few.

☐   There is a distinction between *community-level services*, which aim to improve the well-being for a whole neighbourhood or community, and *community-based services*, which aim to meet the specific needs of individuals and families. They are often closely interlinked and both are part of community practice.

☐   Sound community practice is built on four pillars: building local capacity, focusing on outcomes (not service outputs), preventing the emergence of deep-seated problems for the area and people who live there, and managing local knowledge.

CHAPTER 3

COLLABORATION AND PARTNERSHIP: DELIVERING JOINED-UP SERVICES IN NEIGHBOURHOODS AND COMMUNITIES

OBJECTIVES

By the end of this chapter you should:

- Understand why partnerships are now necessary for delivering integrated, holistic services at local level

- Be familiar with the limitations, difficulties and dilemmas of partnership working which practice, experience and research have uncovered

- Be clear as to the foundations for robust partnerships: trust, sharing information and strong networks

- Be able to take steps towards building 'communities of practice' and consolidating practitioner networks

- Be familiar with methods such as log frames for planning and tracking services across complex partnerships.

Several contemporary pressures make it necessary to solve urgent public problems through intensively negotiated, collaboration-driven, stakeholder-engaged partnerships. Among these are:

- the new orientation of 'enabling' government and more dispersed forms of local governance
- rapid social and economic change putting unprecedented pressures on social environments
- the erosion of historic forms of social connectedness and civic engagement

- dramatic decline in the levels of trust in government and public authorities
- the perceived failure of the conventional top-down, expert-defined, single-organisation approach to finding solutions to social problems.

As a consequence, shaping holistic services is intimately linked to solutions – moving from inadequate, fragmented systems – that will serve families and individuals 'holistically, cost effectively, humanely and creatively' (Briggs 2002: 45). It is only unbounded, prevention-oriented, neighbourhood-wide collaborations that will allow practitioners to tackle deprivation and social exclusion and to shape outcomes for children, young people and older people. Collaborative approaches to neighbourhood problems are the most effective ways to prevent crises in families and to reduce caseloads.

WHY THE OLD SERVICE SILOS ARE NO LONGER UP TO THE TASK

To understand why integrated services are now necessary it is also important to understand why the old system of service silos that dominated public services in the second half of the twentieth century is no longer effective. In the period after 1945 local authority and central government service bureaucracies were designed to solve what were seen as discrete problems through centrally managed programmes: providing decent housing for low-income families, establishing an income safety net, tackling ill-health or juvenile delinquency. The welfare services as constructed then relied on hierarchical organisations staffed by professionals, or 'bureau professionals', each with specialist tasks to undertake. Funding followed this division of labour and only served to bolster these structures. What coordination existed between them relied on senior managers rising above the specialisation and fragmentation.

But in the 1990s awareness of the complexity and sheer intractability of many of the problems besetting society – child poverty, the decline and deprivation of social housing estates, the low level of skills of many young men, community safety, social exclusion of older or disabled people, racism and ethnic divides – became inescapable. What appeared at first to be a set of separate problems that the welfare state would tackle successfully sooner or later were far more interlinked, urgent and entrenched and required all resources, governmental and non governmental, to be drawn on. The first efforts to re-equip services, such as separating the purchasers of services from the providers in the early 1990s, began the blurring of organisational boundaries, a process which later developments only continued. Thus contracting out, privatising services, public–private finance initiatives, devolution and decentralisation, and the transformation of the voluntary sector continued to blur the boundaries between public, private and voluntary sector throughout the 1990s.

To function in this new world what practitioners needed was 'flexible arrangement, constant adaptation, and the savvy blending of expertise and credibility that requires crossing the boundaries of organisations, sector and governance levels' (Snyder *et al.* 2004: 17).

Yet the bureaucracies in which practitioners and service providers work remained stubbornly resistant to change and retained the same features that classic analyses of bureaucracy had identified in the early twentieth century. Max Weber, writing at that time, saw bureaucracies as characterised by:

- a hierarchical division of labour within which each official has a defined competence and is answerable to a superior; work is regulated by supervision;
- salaried staff with a career structure and who therefore are not open to personal gain resulting from their decision;
- work is directed by explicit rules, impersonally applied; decision-making is routinised and is rule-based;
- officials are trained for their function and control access to stored knowledge;
- bureaucracies are 'goal rational' – they will pursue objectives by the most effective means at their disposal (Gerth and Wright Mills 2007).

Little had changed when some eighty years later service bureaucracies encountered the world of joined-up action. Social workers, as 'street-level bureaucrats' had often found themselves in an ambivalent, even poignant position. They were the front-line staff caught between the imperatives of their values that brought them into the work in the first place and the imperatives of working for bureaucratic organisations. Lipsky's concept of the street-level bureaucrat effectively captured the dilemmas and ensnare-ments that organisations used to compel staff to carry out their duties when otherwise they find their own organisation odious (Lipsky 1980; see also Satymurti 1981).

As one of the most astute observers of this need to move beyond traditional silo culture, Xavier de Souza Briggs, has observed, 'It is not that hierarchies or chains of command have disappeared, only that the limits to their usefulness have become more glaring in the past generation' (2002: 44). Flatter organisations, wider networks, multi-disciplinary project-based work, commingling of teams and new channels of participation have all served to show the considerable limitations of that model. UK policy and practice interested in systems change have sought to turn the disconnected specialist units into cross-functional teams and productive collaboration across organisations in order to move further towards what people are looking for, wanting and needing from their social services. The issue, as Briggs put it, is 'How to produce jointly a . . . service or end outcome that was previously the separate responsibility of multiple producers' (Briggs 2002: 44).

JOINING UP THE ACTION: COLLABORATION, ALLIANCES AND PARTNERSHIPS

Working in partnership is central both to overcoming the way the old bureaucratic services do business with the public and to piecing together multi-disciplinary attacks on deep-seated social problems. Since 1997 government has thrown its full weight behind partnership formation rather than market mechanisms or modified bureaucratic hierarchies for delivering improved services. The onrush of partnerships as a vehicle for service delivery can be tracked by a simple statistic: in 1989 the word 'partnership' was used in Parliament 38 times; in 1999 it was used no fewer than 6197 times (Dowling et al. 2004). Whole theories of local government have sprung into being in the wake of this momentous change. Indeed, the concept of 'governance' has come to signify the extent of this change. Services are no longer the product of government, so the argument goes, but of a more diffuse local process that relies on a multiplicity of stakeholders to deliver the services within, crucially, a decentralised system of oversight and accountability.

Many of the government's flagship programmes rest on multi-agency partnerships: New Deal for Communities, neighbourhood renewal, Health Action Zones, Sure Start Children's Centres, crime reduction partnerships, youth referral panels, youth offending teams, intermediate care for older people, the common assessment platforms for children and the single assessment process for older people all require close collaboration across public and voluntary agencies in any one locality. The Crime and Disorder Act 1998, Health Act 2000, and Local Government Act 1999 provided the statutory basis for making some partnerships mandatory and others strongly advised.

No concept, no matter how useful, can receive such an inflation of attention without undergoing a significant loss of precision. The concept of partnership embraces such immense variation in size, composition and ways of working that it has sapped itself of meaning. Local partnerships are often called into being by powerful service agencies simply in order to obtain funding, but then give few pointers as to how the different partners should conduct themselves in going forward and by what process. As a result the concept of partnership is virtually meaningless until attributes of a specific partnership are made clear: what is it for, who does it include, how long is it to last, what resources are at its disposal? Most importantly, what are the decision-making arrangements and what is the balance of power across the contributors?

Yet the logic of partnership or collaboration is irrefutable. The networked nature of our organisational world has brought with it a move away from hierarchy to laterally organised structures. It is not simply about local organisations working together but a complex process of negotiating across a variety of boundaries. Briggs (2002) identifies these boundaries that organisations seeking to form partnerships for social purpose encounter:

- *Boundaries among the major sectors* – public, private (for profit), voluntary (not for profit) – each with different expectations, interests and resources that they bring to any collaborative effort.
- *Boundaries across types of work* – for example youth justice, where values and approaches to the work are not only different one from another but are in direct conflict.
- *Boundaries among types of providers* (producers) – those that provide direct services, those that advocate and provide information, those that coordinate and build knowledge.
- *Boundaries across levels of operation* – highly localised informal resident groups at one end that may not even have a constitution or rules of work, through to formal neighbourhood organisations and organisations that are city-wide, sub-regional, regional and national in their reach.

Most local service partnerships will have to work across all four boundaries; the complexity of managing them is formidable.

BOX 3.1:   THE PARTNERSHIP CONTINUUM

Cooperative relationships are characterized as informal partnerships that share information between independent partners.

Coordinated partnerships have modest organizational structure and more formal relationships between partners but partners retain their own authority. Like task forces, coordinated partnerships develop structures within which partners agree to work together, establish specific roles for partners in a project and emphasize common tasks and channels of communication among partners.

Collaboration involves durable partnerships that unite multiple organizations around a common purpose and require very complex structures and comprehensive planning to accomplish their goals. It suggests an evolving, more dynamic process than partnership. Authority in a collaborative derives from the collaborative structure and the consensus of the partnership

(Flores *et al.* 2005: 110).

BOX 3.2:   DEFINING COLLABORATION

Collaboration occurs when people from different organizations produce something together through joint effort, resources, and decision making, and share ownership of the final product or service

(Linden 2002: 7).

To collaborate is to labour together. Collaborators do not compromise so much as they confer and contribute. Compromise can imply giving up some part of, or conceding, something. The collaborative process is enriched by diversity among the collaborators – diversity of experience, perspectives, values, abilities and interests. Collaboration is a way of working in which power struggles *and* ineffectual politeness are perceived as detrimental to team goals

(Dettmer *et al.* 2001: 7)

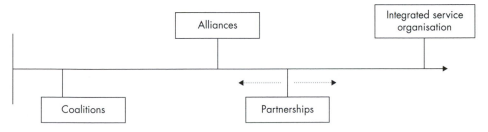

FIGURE 3.1 Continuum from the loosest to the tightest collaborative structures. (Adapated from Roberts 2004)

CONSTRUCTING EFFECTIVE PARTNERSHIPS

The same formula for robust partnerships can be applied to different collaborations but with very different results. Everything depends on how the process is handled. We now have enough accumulated experience of locally based efforts from health and social care, as well as evidence from research, to provide a clearer idea of how to build durable partnerships to promote outcomes for adults and children. Briggs' overview (2002: 21) scopes the following:

- develop standards of success that relate to creating awareness and supportive local attitudes (although relatively intangible) rather than tangible units of service
- choose a base for organising efforts – a neighbourhood, demographic group or profession cluster
- balance this organising with service delivery demands and opportunities and do not let the latter drown out the former
- share leadership and roles of influence as the collaborative constituency building evolves
- bridge class, racial and ethnic divides.

Communication, cooperation and coordination are crucial to success. Differentiated tasks can be allocated among individuals with the various skills to contribute. Sometimes collaboration means recognising differences and finding ways to accommodate those differences. Each partnership should undertake a self-study of preferred styles – reflecting on their own styles and what, as a collaborative, they feel most comfortable with.

BOX 3.3: SIX STEPS IN EFFECTIVE PARTNERSHIP FORMATION

- Determining the need for a cross organisational system by exploring the problem set: What intractable problems have arisen in the environment that *cannot* be resolved by one organisation or another.
- Developing the motivation to collaborate: perceived benefits can push levels of enthusiasm higher.
- Identifying members who care about the problem and are willing to join the collaborative process.
- Collaborative planning: what kind of cross-organisational entity should be set up and what will be its vision and strategies for action.
- Building the partnership: organise the vision and action into a structure, with leadership, communications, policies and procedures for decision-making and implementation.
- Evaluation of the cross organisational entity in terms of outcomes, quality of interaction between partners and satisfaction from users and practitioners.

(Cummings 1984)

Ask the big questions at the beginning

One key to effective formation of a partnership is to ask big questions at the outset and not presume that an excess of goodwill and shared vision will automatically see all problems through. Roberts (2004) has formulated a simple set of questions that establish the feasibility of a collaborative at the outset: Are the individuals and organisations involved willing to commit time and resources to the work *on a long-term basis*? What assets and capability can be exchanged? What will the different organisations involved both provide and expect to receive? What exactly will be the work or activity the collaborative will undertake? What kinds of risks are involved to partners? (Roberts 2004: 41–42).

In this it is essential to move beyond broad descriptions to the *type* of activity – advocacy, direct service provision, facilitating and enabling others, community building. How will this activity serve our users, reach our strategic goals, achieve desired outcomes?

PARTNERSHIPS, POWER AND 'LATERAL LEADERSHIP'

At every stage in the formation of a partnership and in its subsequent activity, power makes its appearance: who has it, what form does it take, and in what circumstances is it exercised? Whether convening and instigating the collaborative, helping to decide which organisations or which individuals will be part of it, assuming the role of host and servicing the collaborative, defining the problem, setting agendas, or coordinating the activity between meetings – all involve organisations and individuals having and using power. How this power is used is intimately linked to the sense of trust and mutuality that may or may not develop within the collaborative. Decisions are being made and power deployed right from the outset. In the early stages of a collaborative it may seem that decisions taken or procedures set do not matter and that to query them is obstructive. But the interests of participants in the collaborative are already at stake and being augmented or sacrificed in this early stage so the more explicit and transparent the foundation stages are, the greater the level of trust and durability of the collaborative.

Broad patterns of the distribution of power quickly emerge. Roberts (2004) for example distinguishes three types of collaborative organisation:

- Authoritarian and hierarchical: where representative power is consolidated in a board of directors which hires a chief executive to oversee activities; members participate through sitting on committees and serving terms on the board.
- Democratic: adopts a participative process, shares information quickly within a network of organisations in order to facilitate innovative decision making.
- Laissez-faire: often convened quickly to respond to an immediate problem and develops haphazardly with little if any structural order.

Thinking about power in community or neighbourhood collaborations

The most common way is to think of power in terms of domination and resistance, of having power and using it or learning how to acquire it. In this sense power is 'power over' others – the thing that allows one person, organisation or nation to compel, pressure, influence, cajole, or coerce other people, groups, organisations, social classes or nations into doing something. This is *instrumental power*, 'something held over you and used to obtain leverage' (Chambers 2004: 25). Power *relations* in this sense are often unequal: those that are dominant pursue their interests and have the power to see that they are realised over those who have less power. Moreover, the structures of a whole society may be so laden with power and the power relations so unequal that the dominant groups rarely have to exercise it in obvious ways since the inequality of power and the coercion is hidden in widely accepted ideas, in the media, in religious faiths and, in family relationships (Edwards and Gaventa 2000). The very fact of inequality in this kind of power may breed resistance through rising social movements, subordinate social classes or political underdogs who seek to develop their own countervailing forms of power in order to even up the balance between 'us' and 'them'. This is a familiar story in history – rebellion, protest, riots and revolution at its most spectacular – but also in other ways: resistance to rape and domestic violence or moves to defend animal rights.

But there is another way of looking at power, one that lends itself more to social work's purposes and methods. A growing number of thinkers (Allen 2003; Chambers 2004) have identified *relational power* or 'associational power', which is exercised with others. This is expressed as the 'power to' rather than 'power over' when people come together to talk and to act. This kind of power provides the capacity to accomplish things that comes from people getting together, discussing, deliberating and reaching agreement on what should be done and how to do it. To nurture this kind of power requires the ability to build relationships and to be able to discuss matters freely in the public square.

Relational power is achieved through recognition of the positive contributions and capabilities of others and nurturing these in others. It is also based on 'self-recognition' – 'the ability to claim our place and space in the world whether others have acknowledged it yet or not' (Chambers 2004: 25). When social work has talked about 'empowerment' it has in general been thinking of power in the first sense – the 'power over' others. But it has done so often in a curiously muted and bloodless way. Empowerment in the social work lexicon has not committed social workers to stiffening the resistance of the oppressed (with some exceptions found in radical social work) but in relatively small gestures around user involvement in some limited areas of decision making (Adams 2003). Yet the second meaning of power affords much greater opportunity for social work to directly apply its skills and knowledge in building local partnerships.

In developing relational power, listening to personal narratives and developing trust and mutual regard are key steps – as they are in the way social work develops relationships and uses self. Often social workers undertake just this but do so in particular ways outlined by the dominant casework paradigm. The same skills can be used for different, wider ends – empowering people, and building collaborative capacity. People want recognition (which is often what the overworked term 'respect' is about) of who they are, what their life story is and what their hopes and fears are. They want to be able to carry forward a meaningful story of their life and to have it validated by others. Moreover, they want the story of their life to help move the 'world as it is' to the 'world as it should be' (Chambers 2004). Social workers have many relationship-building, narrative-forming and listening skills to encourage and develop this hope.

Relational work

In community and neighbourhood practice, values and practice are closely intertwined. Key underlying skills are already embedded in social work and should be familiar to practitioners and students alike. First and foremost is *relational work*. This bedrock skill – forming, maintaining, using relationships – is central to neighbourhood practice. Its uses and purposes are merely extended. Relationships with other professionals, with key participants in a neighbourhood, whether citizens, officers of a local organisation, volunteers, parents or school teachers, are all built on the same basis. Equally social problems are perceived and addressed on a relational basis. As Folgheraiter writes, 'No social problem exists in and of itself; an act of [joint] evaluation is required to make it such' (Folgheraiter 2004: 28). By this he means that perceptions, understandings, moral evaluation and symbolic associations held by many people have to be pooled in order to identify and frame a social problem that requires addressing. Developing and cultivating relationships, often simply in one-to-one relationships, is necessary both to develop effective collaborations and to identify what problems require tackling. The arena is different; the skills remain the same.

BOX 3.4: SOURCES OF POWER

Sources of formal power
- authority vested in positions and titles
- control of scarce resources
- control of structure, rules and regulations
- control of decision-making processes
- control of knowledge and information or expertise
- control of boundaries
- control of technology.

Sources of informal power
- ability to cope with uncertainty
- interpersonal alliances and networks
- systemic power arising from social class, ethnicity, race, gender
- control of symbolism and management of meaning
- control of beliefs and custom
- charisma and confidence
- ability to communicate.

(Adapted from Roberts 2004: 60–61)

ACTIVITY 3.1: WHAT IS THE BALANCE OF POWER WITHIN THE COLLABORATIVE?

Burns and colleagues in their handbook provide a useful exercise to help identify where real power lies – whether in political parties, key professionals and their agencies or members of local communities. Drawing on the results may point to ways of equalising the balance of power over the long term.

On a flip chart create three columns:

- 'Name of organisation or key player'
- 'Rank in power'
- 'Evidence or example of relative power or weakness'.

In the first column list all the organisations or key players involved in the collaborative, including any that you are a member of. Once the list is complete, in the second column rank each in terms of the power they command on a relative scale of 1 to 9, with 9 representing the most powerful and 1 no power. Next to each ranking, in the third column, provide examples that illuminate their powerful or powerless position. The exercise can be conducted within groups, in which case it should begin with a discussion on who the key organisations are with the ranking exercise done by individuals before the group convene again to discuss whether their rankings agree.

(Adapted from Burns *et al.* 2004)

LOCAL AREA AGREEMENTS

Local area agreements have increasingly structured the environment in which partnerships are constructed. They extend and consolidate a process that began several years ago with local area compacts, local public service level agreements and other semi-contractual arrangements that in effect agree to deliver a suite of services to meet local needs. They were introduced on a pilot basis in the spring of 2005 and now in 2007 are national in their implementation. Broadly, a local area agreement is for three years and sets out the priorities for a specific locality negotiated between central government and the local authority, key partners and the Local Strategic Partnership for that area. Four comprehensive areas or blocks are represented in each local area agreement: children and young people, safer and stronger communities, healthier communities and older people, and economic development and enterprise. Additional issues prominent in any given local area and cutting across the four blocks may also be written into the agreement.

Why are local area agreements important to social service practitioners? First, they are outcomes based and seek to deliver those outcomes in ways that are tailored to local concerns and local people. They are particularly responsive to elements of community strategies such as neighbourhood renewal, crime and drugs and children's services. The intention is that increased local discretion and reduced bureaucracy will improve outcomes for local citizens (and reward grants for local authorities) – with a lesser emphasis on stretch targets (ODPM 2005). Of the four blocks only the last one will *not* affect social work and its allied professions. For example, the children and young people's block explicitly embraces the Change for Children agenda and the five outcomes of *Every Child Matters* (see Chapter 5). Agreements reflect the urgency in aggregating local need and looking at existing and future levels of service provision in order to participate in the local area agreement process. While social workers for the local authority or for the large voluntaries may think this is a process that does not involve them, they would in fact be wrong.

Second, there is a process behind each local area agreement in which community engagement and service delivery by the voluntary sector become a critical element in all four blocks. This gives a strong impetus to the 'community-facing' elements of social work, with local people and the voluntary and community sector of the locality drawn into and shaping the process of the design and delivery of the agreement. Guidance is clear that this process should extend beyond ritual forms of involvement to extend to capacity building – that is enhance the pool of skills and knowledge that enable both community organisations and local citizens to make their voice felt in negotiations.

BARRIERS TO GOOD COLLABORATIVE FUNCTIONING

Why do some partnerships work when others do not? The literature from the US and the UK is vast as to why partnerships run into difficulties:

- They are dominated by one or two major agencies that have little real interest in working collaboratively in the sense of sharing power and influence or opening up channels to less influential, more poorly resourced partners to contribute strategy.
- Unprepared partners are hastily brought together to honour the principle of partnership in name only to secure particular project funding.
- Community representatives are often at a disadvantage in terms of knowledge of procedures, as well as being short of time arising from competing family or work commitments. Mothers of young children or people with a disability have found it particularly difficult, for practical reasons such as time or location of meetings, to contribute as they would wish.
- Marginalised groups in the neighbourhood remain excluded because they are overlooked in the partnership formation from the beginning.
- An exaggerated rhetoric of cosiness prevails ('we're all in this together') when in fact decisions are taken elsewhere by a few powerful stakeholders.
- Too much time is spent on 'process', that is in setting up the partnership, in lengthy meetings and in endless consultation with constituent groups, so that there is little sense of concrete achievement.
- The partnership attempts to achieve too much too soon, without sufficient attention to how decisions are made or who has influence (for excellent discussions of these difficult matters see Kubisch *et al.* 1995).

Inter-professional collaboration 'rests on an implicit ideology of neutral benevolent expertise in the service of consensual, self-evident values' (Challis *et al.*: 1988: 17 cited in Easen *et al.* 2000: 356). But different professional groups conceptualise their practice in quite different ways. Evidence shows that partnership working per se does not guarantee positive improvements to services or progress toward outcomes. Often alliances are made up of organisations of hugely uneven capacity and hold vastly different views about deep-seated problems for which 'every solution is value laden, [with] different and shifting organisational interests and elusive performance goals (that have to respond to an ever changing set of community demands)' (Briggs 2002: 49). To work well partnerships require continuous reflection on the collaborative process. In Briggs' phrase, 'Social problem-solving alliances are challenged to pick problems well, develop strategies effectively, and do the hard work of producing smarter [solutions]' (Briggs 2002: 49).

There is another point. Organisations in collaboration are not unencumbered rational actors who are thinking only about users' interests and benefits. Rather their behaviour is shaped by their perception of what the social problem is that the collaboration is intending to tackle as well as by mistrust and information overload. Most community organisations respond to their own stakeholders – funders, regulators, users – and do not believe that cooperation is in their agency's best interest, especially when autonomy and managerial autonomy in particular is threatened or scarce resources are shared (Provan and Milward 2001). Outright manipulation, loss of trust and open dispute can lie behind the tactics of some partners. Many factors make the world of collaboration an imperfect one. No one stakeholder will have a comprehensive view – this is only assembled for the collaborative over time, through negotiation, through putting the jigsaw together (even with pieces missing).

Central government policy has too often implied that partnerships have a commonality of purpose that is in fact not there and seems to suggest that there are no fundamental structural problems to resolve, but have merely to find the right formula for bringing organisations together (Easen *et al.* 2000). This way of presenting the issue hides, as we shall see below, the fact that most collaborations and partnerships actually pit one bureaucracy against another in a fundamental clash of interests. Such unresolved fundamental conflict brings its own difficulties. In an effort to keep all stakeholders satisfied, there is a proliferation of aims and a lack of agreement on ways to achieve them. The number of specialists and consultants used by the partnership may expand. The problem of multiple goals and many stakeholders means that every decision or suggested activity involves a series of trade-offs and compromises within the partnership.

A service organisation's own systems are not necessarily always geared to facilitate smooth collaborative working. The lack of rewards for collaborative skills, individual performance appraisal systems tied to internal technical skills, loyalty in following internal rules and processes, and using resources as directed by senior management all conspire to put a brake on collaborative behaviour by practitioners.

A number of impediments to change arise from these structural arrangements. First, service organisations have nursed internal environments that have a long history of fragmentation, competition and reaction to events, which in turn has fostered emphases on survival, establishing a public image of getting things right, and being seen to exert control over complex situations which in fact require fluidity, and adaptability. Second, there is a failure to grasp the sheer complexity of social structures and how it shapes and sustains social problems. Third, there are, as Bellefeuille and Hemingway starkly put it, 'a plethora of professionals and an industry of care that perpetuates itself in the absence of addressing the fundamental structural problems' (Bellefeuille and Hemingway: 2005: 495).

CASE STUDY 3.1: STREET SEX WORKERS

In one extensive survey on attitudes towards sex workers across five urban neighbourhoods in Glasgow, Staffordshire and elsewhere, Pitcher and her colleagues found that residents held very different views of sex workers' effect on their neighbourhood. For many the presence of sex workers did not affect their overall quality of life yet they had concerns about the visibility of sex work, the impact it had on their use of public space and the association with drugs and crime. They frequently stated that debris, particularly discarded condoms, was all too obvious. The majority view was that sex workers used drugs, and some residents were worried about old needles and drug dealing. These views were linked to wider concerns about personal safety in deprived neighbourhoods with high population turnover, heightened perceptions of risk and crime, disorder and lack of social control. Overall attitudes to sex workers themselves spanned from considerable sympathy and wish to engage with them positively to driving them from the neighbourhood. Sex workers also had fears of violence – from clients but also passers-by – and of low-level abuse (Pitcher et al. 2006).

Local agencies such as the police and local authorities had tried to tackle the public problems through enforcement relying on anti-social behaviour orders (ASBOs) and criminal ASBOs. But this approach proved problematic because it denied women access to vital services, especially drug counselling, sexual health and safer working practices. It also forced them to operate in unsafe areas, increasing their vulnerability. In one neighbourhood ASBOs were used indiscriminately, while in another they were used selectively coupled with 'a practical, non-judgemental view of adult prostitution' (Pitcher et al. 2006).

The drawbacks to wide use of criminal policing became apparent: lack of consistency and blanket restrictiveness resulted in dispersing sex workers to other areas. There were other consequences: media intrusion and public stigma for the whole area. For the individual sex workers it meant criminalisation and lack of support.

This example brings together the different levels of work that a neighbourhood practice requires: being multi-faceted and, multi-agency but working closely with those affected – in this case the sex workers themselves and the residents of the areas in which they work. As a result there are competing demands, competing perspectives and needs and no easy solutions to offer.

ACTIVITY 3.2: SEX WORKERS IN THE LOCALITY: HOW TO RESPOND?

Read the above case study and note some of the practice responses to sex-working in neighbourhoods with their consequences, intended and unintended. Then reflect on what your own position and attitude would be, first as a person resident in an area where sex-working was taking place and second as a practitioner working in a disadvantaged neighbourhood such as those that were the subject of the research.

Would you support the concept of 'tolerance zones' – designated public space for sex-working? Whose interests should come first – that of the sex workers or of local residents? Would you support a multi-agency partnership based on a 'practical, non-judgemental view of adult prostitution'? Should sex-work, and particularly its clients, be subject to greater levels of criminal investigation? Broadly, do you favour greater penalties for sex workers or greater levels of engagement?

SPECIFIC DIFFICULTIES IN HEALTH AND SOCIAL CARE PARTNERSHIPS

Partnerships between health and social care have their own particular difficulties. Hudson (2002) has summarised three important factors in this. First, the training and socialisation of bureau-professions such as housing officers, nursing, and social work establish separate cultures and professional identities that practitioners want to protect. The fact that they often work in common territory can sometimes only accentuate the sense of 'loss of turf'. Second, there are emerging differences in status, and the perceived difference in status can cause a 'matching problem', that is, one group is only willing to work with those of equal status. Third is the matter of professional discretion protecting the freedom to make decisions and to act autonomously, which in social work is valued very highly but sometimes clashes with clinical diagnosticians and the hierarchical cast of the medical profession.

Such marked differences between the ways in which professional groups conceptualised their roles, purposes and practices are frequently attributed to 'cultural' differences between organisations – for example in the way professional expertise is developed through training. As Easen and colleagues noted in their investigations, health visitors with expertise in child health and head teachers came into conflict with community workers whose approach was based on empowering community members; each had a very different view of what 'health work' should be. Head teachers wanted rapid solutions in relation to a particular child whereas social workers focused on longer-term, whole-family solutions (Easen *et al*. 2000).

Research tends to support the notion that the two professions are still in an evolving, indeterminate relationship. Kharicha and colleagues' evaluation of collaborative working between social work and medical practices used six process measures which they studied in some depth: user satisfaction, response time and accessibility, visible collaboration, simplified assessment processes, information transfer and personal care. They reported inconclusive results through the 1990s, finding little shift from examining changes in processes and systems to evaluating outcomes. What outcome studies there were indicated little evidence that collaborative working had made a positive impact on outcomes (Kharicha *et al*. 2004). These issues are examined more closely in relation to services for older people in Chapter seven.

CASE STUDY 3.2:   HEALTH AND SOCIAL CARE COLLABORATION IN NEWCASTLE-UPON-TYNE

In trying to bring some pattern to the tangle of collaborative activity, Easen and colleagues researched two social housing estates in Newcastle-upon-Tyne. They developed two dimensions – 'boundedness' and 'context'. *Boundedness* signifies the extent to which collaborative effort had specified outcomes, timescales and procedures, such as child protection work. *Context* indicates the extent to which collaboration focused on individual users of service or the wider community projects. Collaboration in the latter, less bounded form proved problematic, with conflicting interpretations as to what constituted an intervention, who should carry it out, and with different timescales, different definitions of crisis and different ways of organising services.

Paradoxically, developing a child protection policy for the whole neighbourhood provided a rich example of what happens when several professional orientations try to work in a less bounded context. While there was some scope for sinking professional differences, particularly when working with individual families, the lack of specified outcomes and the continuous need to pursue funding through time-consuming applications undermined mutual goodwill. The failure to release staff from statutory duties further thwarted collaboration (Easen *et al*. 2000).

The conditions in which the practitioners operated also proved critical to collaborative effectiveness in the study. Statutory responsibilities, the availability of time and the particular management structures all played a significant part in setting different, conflicting professional concepts of role and responsibility. However, a sense of shared purpose enabled professional differences to be a creative factor in which a variety of perspectives and resources were brought to bear on a common concern. Crucially, the authors noted the impact of geographical and political factors specific to the localities in shaping practitioner conceptualisation of their work (Easen *et al*. 2000). In the estates they studied there existed already a network of multi-agency contact as well as an existing infrastructure – meeting rooms, funding and inter-agency standing committees – to draw on while other nearby localities had little or nothing (Easen *et al*. 2000).

Easen and colleagues concluded from their research that 'In those professions such as social work which had statutory duties to individual clients but not to community development *per se* it was particularly difficult for the front line managers to make time for their field staff to become involved in community projects or even to do so themselves other than as members of steering/advisory groups' (Easen *et al*. 2000: 362). The practitioners in the Easen study all saw that collaboration focused on the wider locality was required rather than a narrower individual focus. The root causes of social and health problems were unemployment, crime, low educational attainment, absence of social cohesion and the high levels of stress from living in such communities. The tragedy is that they saw what was required but believed they could not change anything.

BUILDING TRUST IN COLLABORATIVE RELATIONSHIPS

Much has been written about trust in the last dozen years, and for good reason: it is the cornerstone of functioning partnership. Partnerships that operate with a high level of trust are more efficient because they enjoy lower oversight and monitoring costs. This enables a clearer focus on outcomes with changes in practice strategies geared to the dynamic of the situation (Goldsmith and Eggers 2004: 128). Low-trust partnerships on the other hand are costly: public officials have to spend huge amounts of time (and money) negotiating, monitoring, enforcing and policing strict, inflexible contract provision.

Contemporary practitioners work in low-trust environments compared to service environments in the past. One reason for this arises from the new fragmented forms of governance and service delivery for programmes in which contracted services call on many providers with competing interests and philosophies about welfare and justice. Building trust among organisations that are competitors is difficult. Sharing information and data often provides a litmus test for the degree of trust within a collaborative relationship. Contracts are another barometer of trust; the more overly specific, tightly drawn and highly detailed they are the more they are testimony to a low-trust service environment. To create trusting collaborative relationships often means having to convert organisations from adversarial to cooperative thinking.

Another reason is the thinning of the old professional order within local authorities as providers of services, which, while positive in some aspects, has meant a loss of a shared ethic. Greater staff mobility is yet another factor – careerism and performance reviews of individuals by senior managers create an edgy environment for practitioners to function within, while changing policy directives and lack of job security also contribute to low-trust environments.

As a way of repairing this situation Charles Sabel developed a concept he called 'studied trust' or 'vigilant trust' (as opposed to 'blind trust' or 'undying loyalty'), which can emerge in environments where mutually suspicious groups redefine their relations and begin to construct a common allegiance. This mutual commitment is achieved through negotiation and is an exercise in organisational autonomy. It supposes that each party might decide after due deliberation to put its trust elsewhere. In this sense it remains vigilant like a democratic compact which requires of parties that they resolve their disputes in ways that do not compromise their autonomy (Sabel 1993). Goal-setting with related targets to mark progress within a partnership at the outset becomes a crucial stage for aligning partnership values and trust building. Often partnership goals are handed down to partnerships by central government and partnerships have to form *after* this stage. Yet goal definition is crucial to continued trusting relationships.

BUILDING PRACTITIONER-CENTRED NETWORKS

A growing accumulation of studies has broadened our understanding of the significance of practitioner networks and provided helpful pointers as to how to form and maintain them. Practitioner networks contain stored energy by clustering relationships around outcomes. They provide space to lower-level employees where face-to-face relationships can be developed and high-trust environments established where none existed before. Without such networks, partnerships are simply creating new, relatively independent bases for an old service practice. Networks achieve their purpose by developing and drawing on 'lateral' relationships among practitioners from different agencies. Such networks can cross organisational boundaries and build trust to accomplish specific public policy goals, meet performance targets or structure flows of information.

Networks foster organisational learning since they provide access to a broader knowledge base and help promote the spread of successful practices (Goldsmith and Eggers 2004). Knowledge sharing becomes a vital tool for integrating networks. An effective cross-organisation knowledge management system can provide a host of benefits: develop new knowledge, develop solutions, enhance learning, build trust. Networks thrive on both *explicit* knowledge and *tacit* knowledge. The former is objective and information oriented: data bases, practice manuals, websites. The latter exists within the heads of employees – developed through experience, gained by practice and applied study. Tacit knowledge produces judgement 'derived from the accumulation of daily exposure to an environment'. It is often the most valuable form of organisational knowledge and is the source of innovation, but it is also the more difficult to capture and transfer and transform into action across a network.

Goldsmith and Eggers observe that most public agencies have difficulty in sharing knowledge – within their organisation or with external partners. This is because officers operate in rule-based systems that reinforce their sense that it is their duty to control access to important information. Hierarchical systems are particularly prone to placing barriers to prevent the dissemination of knowledge. They write that 'the hierarchy trains its armies that information can be misunderstood, or misconstrued and therefore should be provided only in structured ways' (Goldsmith and Eggers 2004: 109). For example, when social workers look at their practice they see a specific field of responsibility, structured by statute and guidance, policy manuals and bureau procedures. This approach has worked well when problems are compartmentalised and solvable through a specific professional domain – taking a child into care or arranging home adaptations for a stroke patient coming out of hospital. But often this is looking through the wrong end of the telescope, making social problems appear circumscribed, discrete, unconnected, even small. For community-level and community-based services a wider, networked perspective is necessary.

Problem solving in networks

There are several reasons why knowledge is not shared:

- not knowing that someone has specific knowledge
- not being prepared to share your knowledge either through lack of trust or fear of loss of power
- not being willing or able to capture tacit knowledge
- not having an interest in other people's knowledge needs (Goldsmith and Eggers 2004: 109).

Knowledge sharing does not just happen but requires an infrastructure and set of routines that promote the transfer of knowledge within the network: meetings, email, co-location, virtual community bulletin boards and web-based seminars all have their part to play. According to Briggs (2002), problem-solving networks need to:

- allow clusters of practitioners and interested stakeholders to learn together what the 'work' of a shared problem really is and how to approach it jointly
- show how interests get mobilised and shaped and re-shaped through the inevitable mix of conflict and cooperation
- show how participants (actors) seek agreement based on their interests and values
- produce mechanisms for planning and decision taking
- specify the network or partnership arrangements specifically enough so that the problems – too big, complex or controversial for any one agency to solve on its own – will be concretely addressed.

From networks to 'communities of practice'

The recently developed concept of 'community of practice' places a name on what is a rapidly spreading tool for an effective further stage in network formation. Communities of practice have been defined as 'groups of people linked by technology and informally bound together by a common mission and passion for a joint enterprise' (Goldsmith and Eggers 2004: 110).

Communities of practice are first and foremost a way of developing and retaining practice knowledge. They operate as social learning systems in which practitioners connect to solve problems, share ideas, set standards, build tools and develop relationships with peers and stakeholders. They can be described as an engaged form of reflective practice that provides a new tool for managing and delivering services in a fast-changing, fluid environment where practitioners need to reach beyond the conventional organisational boundaries to solve problems, share ideas and develop relationships with peers, key partners and the public (Snyder *et al.* 2004).

Several factors are driving the formation of communities of practice: the growing complexity of social problems, the availability of new information and communication technology, and the lack of multi-agency, practitioner networks within local government. This last factor is perhaps the most important. There is now no overarching whole-government mechanism for communication and communities of practice are filling that space.

BOX 3.5: WAYS OF DEVELOPING, SHARING AND RETAINING PRACTICE KNOWLEDGE

1. Working through case scenarios
2. Formation of loose social networks
3. Mentoring
4. Reflection and evaluation by coherent groups of peers

5. Communities of practice: 'Communities of practice are groups of people who share a concern, a set of problems or a passion about a topic or something they do and who deepen their knowledge and expertise in this area by interacting on an ongoing basis'.

(Snyder *et al.* 2004: 17)

Communities of practice bring practitioners together who share a domain of interest, have a commitment to it and have a shared competence. It is the shared interest, commitment and competence which allows them to pursue problem solving and learning within that domain. While the concept can be applied to many different fields – from gang members learning to survive on the street to highly skilled professionals such as surgeons trying to solve a technical problem – our interest here is in the formation of communities of practice by practitioners within the service partnerships providing services for young children, social and health care for older people, or developing less punitive community responses to anti-social behaviour by young people.

Communities of practice place a premium on close person-to-person contact. Members, according to Wenger, engage in joint activities and discussions, help each other work through problems and share information. Interaction is the key – a community of practice does not exist unless the members come together regularly to learn. 'In doing this they build relationships that enable them to learn from each other. Such relationships will be based on consistent, but not necessarily daily, interaction even though they work in different settings and have no formal responsibilities to contact one another' (Wenger 1998).

Communities of practice are more than simply communities of interest or of a shared enthusiasm. They are, Wenger reminds us, *practitioners* who over time develop a shared suite of resources – experiences, stories, cases, tools, ways of addressing recurring problems. They are 'boundary-crossing entities'. They have a domain or set of focal issues that members identify as pertinent.

> The 'community' includes the relationships between members and the nature of the interactions – levels of trust, belonging and reciprocity (give and take) between members. The 'practice' consists of a repertoire of tools, methods, and skills as well as members' learning and innovative activity.
>
> (Wenger 1998: 84)

There is a strong overlap with how a thriving local partnership should function. Communities of practice require structuring and leadership, for example a coordinator who can orchestrate activities, raise issues and solve problems, and connect members. The coordinator should know enough about the practice domain to at least know who should be involved. A support team is also needed to carry out certain functions such as planning initiatives, producing educational activities and arranging technological and communications infrastructure.

ACTIVITY 3.3: PARTNERSHIP IN ACTION

Consider the following case study:

A lone mother is bringing up a son in his mid-teens on her own. They live on a moderate-sized social housing estate on the edge of a well-off city in the northwest of England. The son has harassed two older people in the neighbourhood to the extent that he is being watched by the police. As the behaviour continues the police seek and then obtain an ASBO on the boy. In the meantime the mother obtains a place on a job training scheme – one of only two such places – organised by the neighbourhood management team. She spends three days a week on job placement with the team and one day a week in the local college, where she receives training on administrative and teamwork skills. The constabulary feel very strongly that it is an ill-advised placement, with some senior officers in the force actually quite incensed about it. They think it rewards a parent who is failing to control the behaviour of her child. The local bobby, however, supports the mother. Three weeks after the mother starts her work scheme officers visit her house and arrest her for tampering with her electric meter. She is released that evening when the police admit no such tampering took place. The next day the son is arrested for breaking the conditions of his ASBO: he will be sent to court in two weeks' time.

You are member of the local crime and disorder partnership covering the city representing social services. At your monthly meeting a member of the board passes on to you informally the circumstances relating to this family. You feel strongly that certain wrong steps have been taken in handling this matter. As a member of the partnership you think you have the opportunity to correct a wrong. What steps would you take? Who would you approach and why? What information or other tools would you need to carry this through?

KEY POINTS

This chapter has explored the role that collaboration and partnerships play in delivering community and neighbourhood services. It has:

☐ looked at the difficulties and weaknesses that research on partnerships has revealed

☐ looked at the particular difficulties that health and social care partnerships have experienced in the past

☐ explained the role of trust in building effective partnerships

☐ shown how communities of practice are practitioner networks that share and retain practice knowledge useful to their members.

CHAPTER 4

ENGAGING COMMUNITIES AND NEIGHBOURHOODS

OBJECTIVES

In this chapter we explain why participation by local people is necessary. By the end of the chapter you should:

- Know why high levels of participation by local people and community organisations in service planning and delivery are essential for effective community practice

- Be familiar with tools and approaches for involving local citizens in policy and service decision making including mapping need, utilising networks, facilitating meetings and organising volunteers

- Have to hand established benchmarks of participation.

WHY PARTICIPATION IS NECESSARY

The pressure for engaging communities and neighbourhoods directly in developing and delivering local services has grown enormously from the late 1990s and is now inescapable. While some professionals may still harbour the illusion that public involvement occurs at their invitation, citizen participation in the overseeing and delivery of local services is a necessary segment of practice that cannot be selectively invoked when convenient. One reason for this is that the public at large has changed its attitude toward service providers; it expects to have greater weight in the overall structure and content of services. Professional training no longer provides that mystique of knowledge separating the professional from lay people – instead, the division that does exist is between service practitioners with control over resources and an intelligent citizenry that wants those resources used in a direction of their own making.

A second reason, linked to the first, is the growth of strong advocacy and citizen movements; they hold highly knowledgeable positions and are able to mount public awareness campaigns. There is little choice then but to engage communities for the simple reason that British society is made up of millions of better-informed people, with unprecedented levels of understanding and information who want to apply that knowledge.

Finding and nurturing community representatives

Strong levels of participation provide the foundation for public support of public and voluntary services. It comes through many different channels such as local councillors, user groups or residents' associations or through links with local institutions such as schools, GP surgeries, leisure facilities, faith institutions and libraries. The public may voice opinions at meetings, through questionnaires and surveys, and letters to the editor of the local paper. Shaping services through community engagement has many decision points and should provide many entry points for local citizens to participate. There is no set formula for achieving adequate participation, but the public soon detects when it is mechanistic or done out of duty or as a result of requirement. The challenge for services is, in Xavier de Souza Brigg's fine phrase, to find 'the will and the way' to forms of participation that are useful to local people (Briggs 2002).

Benchmarks for participation

It is important to establish some means by which practitioners, community organisations and local people know whether they are making progress in participatory efforts. One way to do this is through benchmarking. Benchmarks are signposts to help practitioners, managers and local people identify any progress in citizen participation. Important work in the field of regeneration has provided some useful, verifiable benchmarks now recognised to have wide application and that are adaptable to measure the extent of engagement with communities. Benchmarks serve several purposes (Yorkshire Forward 2000):

- they allow progress in participatory initiatives to be tracked
- they raise the profile of community participation and provide the basis for rolling discussion and publicity within the neighbourhood and beyond
- they can form the basis for induction programmes for local people or community representatives who are coming new to a project
- they are central to programme planning from the beginning.

One of the more significant benchmarks in the field, the Active Partners framework developed by COGS for Yorkshire Forward, divides community participation into four dimensions:

Influence: the structures through which local people exert leverage over services, mapping of need, creation of service-level agreements and implementation.

Communication: the degree to which effective ways have been developed that share information, store and retrieve knowledge and devise ways for the incorporation of local knowledge into service planning.

Inclusivity: How all groups with an interest in the locality can participate and the ways in which inequality may be addressed.

Capacity: How local people are provided with the resources sufficient to participate and acquire the skills, knowledge and understanding that allows them to do so effectively (Wilson and Wilde 2003).

Capacity	Communication
How partnerships provide the resources required by communities to participate and support both local people and those from partner agencies to develop their understanding, knowledge and skills. Benchmarks: 1 Communities are resourced to participate. 2 Understanding, knowledge and skills are developed to support partnership working.	How partnerships develop effective ways of sharing information with communities and clear procedures that maximise community participation. Benchmarks: 1 A two-way information strategy is developed and implemented. 2 Programme and project procedures are clear and accessible.
Inclusivity How partnerships ensure all groups and interests in the community can participate, and the ways in which inequality is addressed. Benchmarks: 1 The diversity of local communities and interests is reflected at all levels of the regeneration process. 2 Equal opportunities policies are in place and implemented. 3 Unpaid workers/volunteer activists are valued.	**Influence** How partnerships involve communities in the 'shaping' of regeneration plans/activities and in all decision making. Benchmarks: 1 The community is recognised and valued as an equal partner at all stages of the process. 2 There is meaningful community representation on all decision-making bodies from initiation. 3 All community members have the opportunity to participate. 4 Communities have access to and control over resources. 5 Evaluation of regeneration partnerships incorporates a community agenda. The purpose of the key considerations is to help those using the benchmarks to relate them to their own practice. In answering these questions, partnerships can begin to identify their current position and possible future action.

FIGURE 4.1 Benchmarks for participation: the four dimensions of community participation (from Wilson and Wilde 2003)

Benchmarks such as these are not simply there to provide an annual snapshot of the degree of participation but can be used as a catalyst for bringing clarity to service objectives, and to the process of those services engaging with the community. For this, a workshop for members of community groups and other partners in service delivery can be effective. A facilitator helps the group examine the benchmarks and what they mean, and a discussion follows on what specific indicators or targets would be appropriate for their locality. There is nothing difficult in this: a flip chart and post it notes provided to members, who may be in pairs (or small groups or individually), allow them to chart and record the discussion. The aim is to produce benchmarks – which may or may not follow the four dimensions above – relevant to the local area and to the services involved. This process takes the group into gathering information about a baseline position and to devise actions from the community and/or particular services that would meet those indicators (Wilson and Wilde 2003).

COMMUNITY ENGAGEMENT AND GOVERNMENT POLICY

Government has begun to use the term 'engagement' more frequently in its policy documents and guidance to embrace both *participation* and *empowerment*. As with these related concepts, engagement means different things to different people depending on their point of view. What will appear as a full and fair level of engagement with local people to a local government social worker may well appear thin and tokenistic to an older persons' advocacy group.

Central government has made a strong push for local people to become more actively involved in their neighbourhoods. The best way to get services delivered effectively, it argues, is:

> for local people to take an active role in solving problems. By encouraging local authorities and service providers to give local people more influence over what is delivered and how; and by ensuring that local people have the opportunities, support and tools to get together to drive improvements in their neighbourhoods and in the services delivered to local people.
> (Home Office and ODPM 2005: 6)

The Local Government Act 2000 provided the early legislative basis for community participation in local strategic partnerships, but the phrase 'community engagement' signals a considerable widening of intention and scope on the part of government. Sure Start children's centres, youth referral panels and services for older people and people with disabilities all now put a high premium on involvement. What government wants to see are services more responsive to the wishes and priorities of local communities and more communities taking active control of their own neighbourhoods, including managing their own resources such as playgrounds and community buildings, and establishing their own political authority in the form of parish councils with elected councillors who actively lead. Neighbourhoods are the critical level at which people engage. *Citizen Engagement*, the key strategy document from the Home Office, makes clear that:

• it is critical to clarify whether the purpose of a neighbourhood structure is greater efficiency of service delivery or greater citizen engagement

- successful outcomes depend on a culture change at the centre of the public agencies involved in combination with strong political leadership from the responsible local authority
- neighbourhood management should not be an add-on that marginalises wider civic renewal and fragments the capacity of public agencies to join up wider responses to deprivation
- participatory approaches need to be fit for systematic, long-term participation in neighbourhood structures; these structures need to be efficient – so that local residents make a maximum impact from their involvement.

There is a central tension within *Citizen Engagement* and government strategy for neighbourhood engagement. Government is seeking to drive down costs at the same time as integrating services and focusing service outcomes on major problems as defined by local residents. Yet engaging communities and neighbourhoods is a long-haul task with many obstacles along the way. 'Local people' may turn out to be few in number and already overburdened with participative responsibilities in other initiatives. Workshops can get bogged down, the process extend out in time, the neighbourhood may be extremely diverse in perspective, sparking resentment and opposition among different local groups, personalities can be contentious and disruptive, and there may be a shortfall of skills or will or both. This is what comes with the territory; it is what happens when genuine choices open up, when opportunities arise for local people to exert real influence, perhaps for the first time in their lives.

BOX 4.1: BLACON NEIGHBOURHOOD MANAGEMENT COMMUNITY ENGAGEMENT CHECKLIST

The Blacon community engagement checklist places a responsibility upon all working in the Blacon area to ensure that consultations, policies and services observe the requirements of the checklist. It embraces four interlocking levels of community engagement – strategic/board level, organisational/management level, operational/delivery level and community level. The aim of the checklist is to ensure effective participation of Blacon residents and emphasises the creative possibilities of the community working collaboratively with key health, justice and social welfare agencies. (This checklist is available from the Blacon Neighbourhood Management Pathfinder. The excerpt below omits the section on strategic and board level work for reasons of space.)

Organisational level
- Determine what your community engagement principles are.
- Profile the community – its composition, needs, concerns and resources.
- Undertake a 'stakeholder analysis', that is determine which groups, organisations or individuals need to be involved and establish a key stakeholder group to contribute to the detailed design, implementation and evaluation of the strategy.
- Ensure that all those involved understand what the strategy is trying to achieve.

continued

- Identify training and support needs for staff and volunteers.
- Select appropriate tools that will facilitate community engagement.
- Decide operational priorities in the context of resources.
- Identify barriers to engagement and ways of overcoming them.
- Produce a detailed action plan for implementing the strategy and establish ways of giving feedback on progress to the community.

Operational/practitioner level
- Ensure you understand your role and responsibilities in engaging the community.
- Consider what changes you may need to make in how you work, taking account of the community engagement principles.
- Make sure you have the time, resources and support to do what's being asked of you.
- Identify training and support needs you may have.
- Get to know the community you are working with and listen to what people are saying about its needs and concerns.
- Let people know what it is you are trying to do.
- Identify ways in which the community can meaningfully influence the services you are delivering.
- Tell the community about the difference people can make by getting involved but make sure you get the balance right between encouraging aspirations without raising false expectations.

Community level
- Find out why community engagement is happening – what is the bigger picture?
- What is the nature of the commitment from service agencies – is it genuine?
- Has the community been consulted over the amount of involvement it would like?
- In what ways are community representatives accountable?
- Is there sufficient practical support to ensure full citizen participation?
- Has the community had the opportunity to contribute to decision making?
- Is the community involved in evaluation of implementation of any plans?

(Adapted from the Blacon Neighbourhood Management Pathfinder, 2005)

Empowerment

Empowering others, according to Ciulla, means doing one of the following: 'you help [people] recognize the power that they already have, you recover power that they once had and lost, or you give them power that they never had before' (Ciulla 2004: 60). She argues that authentic empowerment entails a distinct set of moral understandings and commitments between those leading the process and those being empowered. The moral concepts she has in mind are responsibility, trust, respect and loyalty. They are reciprocal, 'that is, they exist only if they are part of the relationship between followers and leaders'.

> When leaders really empower people they give them the responsibility that comes with that power. Empowerment programs that give employees

responsibility without control are cruel and stressful. Authentic empowerment gives employees control over outcomes so that they can be responsible for their work.

(Ciulla 2004: 78)

Social work and the broader world of social care has for two decades and more explored ways of empowering service users, whether individuals or in groups. Across that time there have been bold explorations as to what empowerment means, particularly in relation to people who are oppressed, whether through racism, domestic violence, barriers for disabled people, or all forms of keeping certain groups of people subordinate and intimidated (Dalrymple and Burke 1995).

Alongside this exploration of empowerment there has been healthy scepticism within the profession as to what the concept actually means in the context of social service. 'Empowerment', Mullender and Ward wrote, 'is used to justify propositions, which at root represent varying ideological and political positions . . . which lack specificity and gloss over significant differences' (Mullender and Ward 1991: 1). The ambiguity of meaning for terms like empowerment and participation has become even greater in the era of partnerships and collaborative working where local people are being invited to take up positions of influence in the face of multi-disciplinary cross-professional networks.

The recent policy emphasis on the involvement of local people in designing, managing and monitoring neighbourhood-based initiatives of all kinds has brought both unprecedented opportunities and pressure on their time, skills and resources. Community members are now required to be consulted about how considerable sums of government money are to be spent and are expected to provide representation on steering groups, management boards and neighbourhood forums of many kinds. They are expected to put their minds and efforts to solving difficult local problems such as drug abuse, anti-social behaviour and care for older people.

Local people, especially those who are volunteering their time and effort, want to put trust in these partnership arrangements. However, there is often conflict between the rhetoric of partnership coming from those holding power and this sense of trust. This is why bogus empowerment is so devastating. Residents can feel foolish about falling for inflated claims and undelivered promises, while partnership leaders lose credibility and respect because they have blatantly failed to show commitment to the partnership's ideals.

Problems with engaging citizens in disadvantaged neighbourhoods

Citizens of lower social and economic status are at a disadvantage when it comes to participating in local affairs. They have to struggle against experiences that tell them that government is really not much concerned with their interests and aspirations and that the public sphere is open to citizens 'by invitation only' (Schier 2000). Voluminous studies on participation in the US have shown the disparity in levels of participative activity according to income (Verba et al. 1995). The public sphere at all levels and across all sectors, is dominated by upper income bracket professionals possessing specialised knowledge who understand the process and the coded language through which public points are made to stick. They in turn are backed by organised interest groups capable of marshalling impressive amounts of money and expertise to bend policy their way (Markus 2002).

Social agencies including social workers have played an ambiguous role in empowering and participative process. They have frequently disempowered local people instead through their 'disabling help'. Distancing from and even distrust of services arise not only through the low expectations of what those services can provide but through the narrow range of choices that come with living in an area dominated by poor services, which makes people all too aware of their difficulty in accessing the things in life which will help them realise their own aspirations. Xavier de Souza Briggs writes: 'There is no such thing [as apathy]. People are not used to participating, they are not used to wielding any kind of significant influence. They are used to turning out for two hour meetings of which the first hour and three quarters consist of a presentation of plans for services in the locality and the last 15 minutes are for questions' (Briggs 2002: 7).

APPROACHES TO COMMUNITY ENGAGEMENT

There are a number of models and approaches to engaging communities in delivering community-level services or community-based services (for definitions of these terms see Chapter 2).

Community development

Community development approaches have expanded enormously since the late 1990s in part because of the range of government initiatives incorporating community-level objectives with funding attached. Whereas in the 1970s community development would have been the remit of free-floating community workers, now 'community development workers' are often attached to specific services – Sure Starts, neighbourhood management schemes, community arts, health promotion initiatives, youth work, and local anti-drug campaigns.

Community development work is a form of capacity building (see Chapter 2). It aims to galvanise local people to debate the issues of most concern and then to enable them to cohere around a feasible programme of action that will effect the change required to deal with the identified problem. Radical community development 'provides a starting point for linking knowledge to power and a commitment to developing forms of community life that take seriously the struggle for democracy and social justice' (MacLaren, 1995: 34, cited in Ledwith 2005).

The Brazilian educationist Paolo Freire has had a huge impact in the way community development has been seen as an educative process. He argued that perceptions of powerlessness erode hope and create a 'culture of silence', which goes some way to explaining why the poor seem to accept the harshness of their lives and settle for explanations of individual failure rather than collective oppression.

Freire believed that every human being is capable of critically engaging with their world once they begin to question the contradictions that shape their lives through a process of what he called 'conscientisation' – the process of becoming aware of contradictions, whether political, cultural or socio-economic. The worker seeks to draw out from people's experiences what the most pressing problems are and to 'problematise' them, i.e. look at the complexity and their relationship to forces well beyond the power of the individual to change on their own. Freire promoted a 'critical pedagogy' through which every process of community organising has to contain a process of education. Education cannot be neutral: either it serves the *reproduction* of the dominant order or provides space for *production* in which citizens learn to think for themselves. Such a pedagogy should include the basic skill of dialogue – a mutual and reciprocal form of communication that embodies respect – and acknowledges the importance of relationship. Without this community development work would only begin to recreate another, albeit different system which would impose its own values, assumptions, perceptions. (For an excellent discussion of Freire's continuing relevance see Ledwith 2005.)

ACTIVITY 4.1: STRATEGY CHART

Aims	Constituents, allies & opponents	Targets	Approaches & tactics
Long-term objectives Intermediate goals	Whose problem is it? Who cares about this issue enough to join in? Who gains if goals are attained? Who are the opponents?	Who has the power to give you what you want? (Maybe a person, a decision, an institution) How can they be persuaded to help achieve your objective?	What approaches will you use? What negotiations do you need to enter into and over what? Who will you contact? What arguments or claims will be made?

FIGURE 4.2 Strategy chart (adapted from Bobo *et al.* 2000)

While you may be unfamiliar or even uneasy with using the community development approach you may have more of a 'community level' or community development role than you might think. Consider any initiatives, campaigns or even one-off actions that you are participating in and lay them out within the chart framework. Does it help clarify your intervention?

Community learning

The term 'community learning' embraces a wide number of initiatives that combine education with efforts to increase citizen involvement in local affairs. Family learning in community schools, bringing in local people to help design children's wards or older people's wards in new or renovated hospitals, involving young people in landscaping derelict urban land, young people's parish councils, dance projects with hearing impaired people, football and sports programmes for excluded youth, community theatre projects headed by disabled people, parent education classes and Asian women acquiring computer skills are all examples of community learning. Such initiatives are rapidly multiplying and are often unsung and even unknown in a given locality. Making an inventory of such projects and linking with them where relevant is an important step in finding potential partners for community-level initiatives.

Many of the techniques of adult education are spreading outward from their previous deployment in evening classes and formal adult learning settings into more informal learning. There are a number of ways to think about how to construct learning situations that are sociable, practical and creative. Local residents are much more likely to become engaged in learning if they are enjoying themselves and if they can see results. Learning that is responsive and engaging will:

- build on what people know from their own experience and everyday lives
- draw on local expertise
- encourage people to learn from each other and with each other
- introduce new knowledge and skills when appropriate
- base teaching on methods that are participatory, interactive, practical and creative
- aim at problem solving and critical thinking about people's experiences and social and familial situations
- be based on teachers who are able to establish equal and respectful relationships with learners and who are sensitive to cultural and religious differences (Thompson 2002).

Neighbourhood forums

These have spread widely with the development of neighbourhood management approaches and have acquired a broad range of functions, both formal and informal. As part of a formal neighbourhood services collaborative they provide resident memberships focusing on particular issues, concerns or services such as community safety, education, early years services or social care for vulnerable adults. The forums are often chaired by a resident and mix residents and community organisation representatives with local officials as members. They conduct their own deliberations and evaluations and provide local knowledge and reach decisions which are then fed into board meetings or collaborative policy.

As informal mechanisms forums may be convened at regular intervals around a particular theme or sector. Forums are characterised by their stability and relative longevity. They may be part of a devolution initiative organised by the local authority or in fact arise from the community itself as it begins to involve itself in partnerships or other collaboratives (see Chapter 3). If the former they may have limited decision-making powers (or none) but if the latter they may acquire an important seat 'at the table' with their voice growing progressively more important as the neighbourhood initiative matures.

The strength of neighbourhood forums are their:

- regular long-term contacts with a consistent membership
- capacity to build trust and mutual understanding and nurture new ideas over time
- ability to consider issues in depth and at a strategic level
- low running costs.

To bring these out requires a good facilitator, an explicit purpose and even, if the forum is large, sub-groups to take particular topics forward.

On the other hand their weaknesses can be:

- the ambiguity of their remit – do they have decision-making powers or are they simply consultative?
- their relatively small membership – vulnerable to absenteeism or a falling off of commitment
- if created by the local authority they will usually require substantial servicing (Blacon Neighbourhood Management Pathfinder 2005).

Neighbourhood service agreements

Considerable effort has been devoted to developing local agreements or 'compacts' between the voluntary and community sector and the local authority, which are a framework of principles and processes giving shape to the relationships between these sectors. Essentially these seek to establish who will provide, across these sectors, what services and with what objectives in a given locality. Compacts, while not given legal status, provide another means by which coordination can be achieved and energised; they draw on the enabling powers of the local authority and the project ingenuity and grass roots ties of voluntary and community groups. Certain factors have predisposed some compacts to greater success than others:

- a local history of dialogue between the voluntary and community sectors and the local authority
- a well-supported voluntary and community sector infrastructure which reflects the views of its different elements, in particular smaller, wholly volunteer projects and those from black and Asian communities
- the process of reaching agreement being viewed as an important stage in its own right towards greater mutual understanding (Craig *et al.* 2005).

But in this process it has become clear that black and minority ethnic organisations are at a disadvantage, whether in relation to compacts or any other local agreements. In particular black and minority ethnic voluntary and community organisations feel often marginal to local policy debates and that they are being used by both the larger voluntary sector organisations and the local authority to deliver on their targets (particularly to do with race and ethnicity). This they view as a limited, instrumental role which precludes them from being involved in policy discussions or setting strategic direction for a locality, despite having strong community links and proven records of working in the community (Craig *et al.* 2005).

Reaching an agreement as a process, however, can be productive by clarifying roles and relationships and building a shared framework of understanding between the different sectors (Craig *et al.* 2005). Productive tools for this include learning more of each other's perspectives by role playing 'switching seats at the table', using case studies and 'creative reframing', where problems are deliberately cast in a different framework (Kaner *et al.* 1996: 200–201).

PRACTITIONER SKILLS AND APPROACHES

Facilitation

The new service environment, built on collaboration and partnership, citizen engagement and participation, requires different roles and skills. Broadly these stem from the social worker as *intermediary*. Because they are placed near or at service boundaries, facilitating and mediating between service interests and local people have become critical functions.

The service agency's capacity to draw out and utilise the knowledge, motivation and viewpoints of local citizens is a prerequisite for community's feeling of owner-ship and having a stake in neighbourhood-based services. Facilitation is a key skill for achieving this. While most practitioners will have heard of facilitation, it remains underused even in arenas where participatory decision making is, in theory, supposed to be happening.

Facilitation is different from mediation because it aims to solve dysfunctional conflicts with community groups. More than this it aims to explore complexity and achieve better thinking and clearer positions on matters considered important by local citizens. Facilitation focuses on getting the optimum process in place for participatory group decision making. Facilitation aims to overcome the flaws that dominate group decision making and so stifle creative decision making and create conflict. Flaws typically encountered in local groups include:

- value judgements that inhibit spontaneity and deter others from expressing their views on matters significant to them
- exploration of complexity being discouraged
- emphatically expressed views holding greater sway in a public discussion than tentative or awkwardly put views
- rushed action plans and tight deadlines answering the need to be seen to do something
- considered, deliberative thinking being ignored as counterproductive (Kaner *et al.* 1996).

Participatory groups respond to these problems. Opposing viewpoints are given time and space and are allowed to coexist; people are supportive and draw each other out ('is this what you mean?'); people listen to the ideas of others because they know their own ideas will be heard; members of the group can accurately represent each other's points of view – even if they disagree with them; when the group reaches a decision it reflects a wide range of perspectives. The facilitator encourages everyone to do their best thinking (Kaner *et al.* 1996).

The process a group goes through to solve a new difficult problem is neither smooth nor sequential but often characterised by confusion and misunderstanding. Groups find it difficult to tolerate the ambiguity and conflict that arise when group members do not have shared frames of reference. Yet a group's most significant breakthroughs are often preceded by a period of struggle. A facilitator is often essential to help a group through the awkward, uncomfortable but normal dynamics of working through diverse and conflicting opinions (Kaner *et al.* 1996).

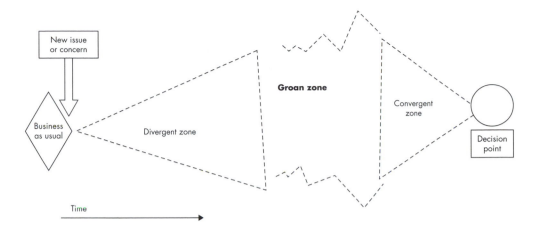

FIGURE 4.3 Diamond of participatory decision making (Kaner *et al.* 1996)

Knowing there is nothing straightforward about group decision-making processes, the role of the facilitator is to help the group overcome a basic problem – that people do not say what they are really thinking. Often comments are likely to be antagonistic or dismissive such as:

- haven't we already covered that point?
- let's keep it simple – please
- we're running out of time
- what does that have to do with anything?
- impossible. Won't work, no way
- I don't want to go there; the days are long gone when that was possible.

Such dismissive comments pressurise others to engage in self-censorship because they want to avoid being put down in this way. The effective facilitator reduces self-censorship to a minimum and bolsters each participant's confidence in their own views.

Public meetings

This is perhaps the oldest and most familiar mode of community engagement for practitioners. Public meetings are preceded by some (usually local) publicity with a general call for attendance. If there is an extremely contentious issue to be dealt with this may spark a large turnout. If the meeting is following the usual format practitioners and managers will have drawn up an agenda already and will sit at a top table facing the audience. The format is familiar to officials and it is often a one-off, relatively easy to organise and low cost.

ACTIVITY 4.2: PUBLIC MEETINGS: SOME DRAWBACKS

Think of a public meeting that you have either attended or helped organise. Which of the following drawbacks did you observe:

• low attendance
• discussion from the floor dominated by a few individuals
• a sizeable majority of the audience remained silent
• presentation from officers and experts took up most of the time
• confrontation between members of the audience and officials at the top table
• sections of the community not present/felt excluded
• attempts at drawing up a 'sense of the meeting' were ineffective?

While the drawbacks of large open meetings often outweigh the gains, smaller, more focused meetings built on pre-existing relationships or meetings convened by specific groups with a specific agenda for deliberation and consultation can be highly effective. Layout of the meeting room can be more informal, smaller discussion groups can be set up allowing a greater number to contribute, and action lists developed.

Running public meetings*

Meetings can make or break any initiative in engaging communities, and bad meetings can finish them off altogether. The sense of wasted time, of overly complicated or dry agendas, of being given the feeling that attendance is for show or for some unknown purpose, of being spoken down to, of it becoming progressively clear that the invited public has no real future role and never will – all can produce pent up feelings of uselessness and antagonism towards the initiative.

Every meeting should push the community engagement initiative forward in one way or another – making decisions, recruiting volunteers, training the board to function more effectively, raising the public's voice, impressing local officials and elected members or telling a story or point of view for the media.

Most meetings are at fault before they have even begun through lack of planning. Effective meetings require careful, at times lengthy, preparation. To fling an agenda together may work with colleagues down the corridor but it will severely hamper a relationship with the public. Careful judgements have to be made as to what issues should surface in the agenda. Each item or proposal should have someone to explain what is at stake. What the role of chair should be, and how and by what means the meeting will reach its decision, should be dealt with in advance. The ways of handling disagreement and open conflict should also be worked through. Finally, agreement about how to communicate the meeting's outcomes to the public at large should be reached in advance.

---

* For this section I am heavily indebted to a particular manual, *Organizing for Change* by Bobo *et al.* 2000. It has helped me clarify how to run effective meetings – and by deduction explain why I have sat through so many bad ones.

- Choosing the right site is also crucial: are people familiar and comfortable with it? Is it accessible for all? What is the symbolic importance for residents (for example a mosque or all-white church, or a community hall the use of which is heavily dominated by a particular organisation)? Are there adequate facilities with scope for a signing-in table (to get all names and addresses) and any necessary equipment in place?
- Child care, transportation and language are all well-known inhibitors to attendance – they have to be thought through well in advance and people have to have trust and confidence in the arrangements. If it is a large meeting some indicator of the quality of the child care and the sensitivity to cultural or faith issues should be given – 'games and activities for even the youngest children' or 'there will be facilities available for prayer during the meeting'.
- Date and time: the meeting must be set for when it is most convenient for those whom you want to attend.
- Agendas should be printed in advance with all participants receiving a copy; each agenda item should have the objective of the discussion on that item and what alternatives there might be, and have suggested time limits for discussion to give an indication of the relative importance of each item.
- Turnout – make plans for reminding people and do as much of that face to face or over the telephone as possible. Explain the important issues and why it is critical to attend the meeting.

CASE STUDY 4.1: A GOOD MEETING GOES BAD

Several years ago a Wave 3 Sure Start was trying to get off the ground in a disadvantaged estate on the edge of a large old industrial city. A public meeting to consult parents and local people was called and on the night there was a large and exemplary turnout in the local community centre. Part of the publicity for the meeting included the invitation to parents to bring their young children and leave them in the playgroup running in an adjacent room.

Unbeknownst to the organisers of the meeting, inspectors had decided to do a spot check on the playgroup at the same time. A parent who had gone into the playgroup to check on her young child saw them arrive and immediately returned to the public meeting with the news that 'social services have come into the playgroup next door'. The hall emptied almost immediately as parents picked up their toddlers and headed for home.

Facilitating a meeting

Facilitating skills are particularly useful in meetings where people are uncertain of one another, where contentious issues and personalities may be prominent or where people lack confidence to put forward their point of view. Facilitating a meeting requires someone who:

- understands the aims of the meeting and each of the individual agenda points
- can keep the meeting on its agenda, to time, and manage the discussion in a way that makes people feel progress is being made towards a decision, outcome and action
- involves everyone in the meeting, ensuring the dominating do not dominate and that the reticent are encouraged to have their say
- ensures decisions are made democratically (Bobo *et al.* 2000).

Virtually all meetings have their 'awkward squad' – those who want to argue or engage in conflict, berate and denigrate, dominate the floor or talk irrelevancies. In dealing with them there are a few retorts to have in mind when facing provocative or unruly behaviour:

- 'This is the agenda: this is what we are here for and this is what we are going to do.'
- 'If you have your own issue – by all means say it; if it doesn't fit with the agenda we will park it – not ignore it – by writing it down on a flip chart and then follow it up. But we can't discuss it tonight.' The fact that it is recognised and written down often meets the sense of urgency that the speaker brings.
- 'Does anyone think they are here for other reasons?' (all from Bobo *et al.* 2000).

ACTIVITY 4.3: HOW TO GUARANTEE A POOR MEETING

Drawing on your experience from attending meetings, reflect with a colleague on why each of the points below are likely to produce an ineffective meeting.

- Time the agenda down to the minute and assume the meeting will start exactly on time.
- Assume that everybody will know what you're trying to accomplish at the meeting – and if they don't they will ask.
- Plan to spend the first half of the meeting prioritising what to do in the second half of the meeting
- Keep the meeting interesting by making sure the people who give reports use overheads and pie charts.
- If you've got an agenda of difficult and important items, improve efficiency by skipping breaks and shortening lunch.
- Save the most important discussion for last, especially if it is emotionally fraught.
- When you know the agenda is too packed, assume the meeting will run overtime but don't tell anyone.
- Don't waste time planning an agenda. Things never go the way you expect them to.

(Adapted from Kaner *et al.* 1996)

OTHER MEANS OF INVOLVING LOCAL PEOPLE

Exhibitions

Exhibitions can often be used to present detailed proposals or suggested innovations. If unstaffed they provide little opportunity to gather comments or answer relevant questions from those who attend. It may also be difficult to summarise opinion from those who attend.

But exhibitions have several potential advantages. While their primary purpose is to convey information to the public they can also be used as a consultative device. The ready availability of large-scale maps combined with digital photography make it possible for even the smallest team to put together a display centred on a few streets and to explore issues that have a spatial concern. A proven technique is to engage people by asking them where they live on the map or whether they can place one or more of the photographs in their community; this can often be a prelude to sounding out their opinions about services or living in the neighbourhood. A further step would be to make the exhibition interactive in the sense that people could be invited to take their own photographs of problem areas or otherwise log concerns within the exhibition itself.

Questionnaires and interviews

Questionnaires and interviews may be conducted or distributed at specific locations, door to door or even over the telephone (using trained interviewers). If properly designed they produce a valuable database that can be compared or integrated with existing data sets as well as analysed with statistical software packages and presented graphically in publications. To be useful in this way questionnaires or interviews need to be designed by experts (which of course can happen in consultation with the public). Informal questionnaires designed by practitioners themselves or members of the community may simply be seeking a rough snapshot of community opinion that does not require the rigour of sampling techniques. With postal questionnaires, rates of return are very low; in any format language barriers and uncertainty over the uses to which a questionnaire will be put often skew the results. The Neighbourhood Management Pathfinder in Blacon, near Chester, stresses that in preparing a questionnaire practitioners should:

- ask why it is being done and how the results will be used
- always involve local groups in the design, collation and analysis
- not jump directly from analysis of results to proposed solutions to social problems.

Smaller communities of place or interest will likely yield better results than a larger, diverse or fragmented community.

Focus groups

Focus groups are small groups of roughly 8 to 10 people who can be either randomly selected or who are representative of wider groups in the community such as older people, parents with young children or young people not in work or education. They are convened on a one off basis to consider carefully structured questions. Although a major marketing tool, focus groups are extremely important vehicles for eliciting a range of opinion, particularly from marginalised groups who may have encountered a range of exclusionary barriers in other forms of opinion giving. They are not, however, decision-making bodies per se. They also require some skill in setting up. There are some parallels with 'citizen juries'.

Pinboard questionnaires

Pinboards are simple to use and easy to understand, perhaps with only a single facilitator to explain how they work. They are also cheap, lightweight and versatile, being pieces of foam board or card on which basis choices or questions are defined. Like basic questionnaires they work best with clear, closed questions requiring a yes or no or choosing options X or Y. Participants are asked to stick a pin or a sticky dot or pen mark next to the category of their choice. They are cheap, active and fun to complete, and are open to all with contributors remaining anonymous. Results accumulate instantly and are visually immediately recognisable. Pictures can be used instead of words if literacy or language familiarity is an issue. The pinboards can be specific to particular groups if required – young, old, male, female, settled population or new arrivals. Choices, however, are often straightforward with little chance for contributors to come forward with new or complex suggestions or ideas. In that sense they are excellent as a supplement to qualitative information already gathered rather than as a stand alone device (Blacon Neighbourhood Management Pathfinder 2005).

LOG FRAMES

The logical framework analysis, or log frame for short, provides an important way to bring partners together at an early stage to develop strategy and then to work through the consequences of that strategy. Log frames exist in time and those who participate in their formation have to work back from the strategic outcomes that they envisage five years in the future to thinking what has to be done in each year preceding in order to achieve those outcomes. The log frame is ultimately a visual map charting the interrelationships between goals and action.

- The log frame identifies the project's goals and allocates measurable and/or tangible performance targets to them.
- It also identifies the inputs and outputs the project will deliver to enable achievement of the proposed goals.
- It finally presents a cause and effect matrix where inputs lead to outputs and outputs lead to immediate objectives, which in turn lead to longer-term goals.

Key components of a log frame

The design summary provides information on the basic building blocks of the project and presents them as a cause–effect chain drawn from a preceding cause–effect analysis. The *inputs* are expected to result in the *outputs*, which in turn are expected to achieve the immediate objective of the project which contributes to the longer term objectives (sometimes called the *goals* of the project.)

	Design summary	Performance targets and indicators	Verification and monitoring mechanisms	Assumptions and risk
Goal (long-term objectives)				
Purpose (immediate objectives)				
Outcomes				
Activities				

FIGURE 4.4 Log frame matrix

Log frame process

The concept of logical framework analysis or log frame has provided a useful tool for all levels of the programme including project workers, managers and board members to identify the role they play within the programme and define the purpose of that contribution. The idea of the log frame is to help partners develop a well-designed but realistic programme and ensures that partners plan, monitor and report on the basis of results. When completed it essentially gives a concise description of the project, demonstrating the relationship between the project's resources, its goals and expected results. Typically it is a results-based project management tool that enables the identification and management of risks while bearing in mind expected results.

CASE STUDY 4.2: LOG FRAME ANALYSIS AT SURE START BLURTON, STOKE-ON-TRENT

Sure Start Blurton used the log frame in a somewhat different way: not for purposes of performance management but as a visionary tool, establishing what its aims were and where it wanted to go. Across a year, from January to December 2003, in a series of workshops guided by academics and practitioners experienced in using log frames, project workers, managers and board members put together a strategic vision of what they wanted the Sure Start to achieve and to establish an agreed account of why it is doing what it is doing.

The role of parent board members, who wanted a clearer sense of direction for the programme, was critical to the success of the process. The parent board members urged that the goal of the programme should not only include the national Sure Start objectives but should also embrace the well-being of communities measured by quality of life indicators. It was parent board members who pressed for strengthening the log frame by re-committing the programme to promoting community capacity by 'improving skills and capacity, community well being, changing service delivery, continuous improvement' (Pierson *et al.* 2004: 32).

For Sure Start project workers the log frame process was not about adding additional tasks or establishing performance indicators. Piecing together the log frames enabled each practitioner to identify how they fit in to specific projects. The completed log frame became a central reference point, providing a clear story for practitioners and others to refer to, one that both located their specific contribution to the overall mission and projected the twelve major themes of the programme.

In all the completed log frame, which fits on a single sheet of A3 paper, outlined twelve themes – each of which is associated with specific projects and which in effect became the key performance targets for the next twelve months. The national public service agreement targets were included but were linked strategically to pathways of activities that the board had identified and were owned by the entire programme. Among these was the significant commitment to a target of 80 per cent of Blurton families recognising and accepting Sure Start Blurton as a 'needs-led service'.

USING VOLUNTEERS

Volunteers are now widely used in a range of settings: parent mentors, youth work, day centres for older people, early years play groups, school pupils mentoring peers and credit unions. Volunteers also give enormous amounts of time and energy to taking part in executive boards of neighbourhood initiatives such as Sure Start Children Centres, neighbourhood management pathfinders and neighbourhood or community forums of all descriptions. Some national organisations build their services around what their volunteers, all of whom have been trained to a uniform high level, have to offer: Home Start provides parent mentoring, Citizens Advice Bureau offers advice on benefits, Age Concern provides services for older people.

Social work as a professionalised activity has only relatively recently embraced the positive role that volunteers play, both in the peer-level expertise they have to offer and the role they play in providing social 'glue' in the locality. The first wave of radical social work in the 1970s was somewhat suspicious of volunteers, who it saw as undermining wages and trade union solidarity. On the other hand community social work as envisioned in the 1980s began explicitly to acknowledge the role for volunteers. In the twenty-first century it is clear that the ensemble of social work activities could not be carried out without volunteers. An emphasis on neighbourhood work means that the use of volunteers should become even more systematic.

- Volunteering provides individuals with a means of expressing values that are important to them. Recruitment to support a specific cause or service within the programme might have greater appeal. It is probably a mistake to couch the encouragement of volunteering only in the context of 'work-readiness' or tackling 'workless households' although it may have that longer-term effect for individuals.
- Recruitment and retention of volunteers go together. Poor recruitment practices lead to increased turnover. To aid recruitment meaningful job assignments could be prepared – with some specification of skill level. There should be some matching of would-be volunteers to specific skills that need to be developed for those particular projects.
- Many first-time volunteers have lofty expectations of what the experience will be like – and so some work around managing those expectations is worthwhile. Volunteers placed in inappropriate jobs will be dissatisfied and quit. Volunteers recruited ineffectively may then form the wrong impression of the organisation and spread this by word of mouth.
- Widen the number of projects that rely on volunteer workers and provide them with the responsibility to seek out and recruit volunteers. Virtually everyone in the service programme should see recruitment as part of their duties. Facilitate the connections between those already serving as volunteers and those who might do so. Current volunteers may provide friends or contacts who they can recruit and then offer support (both emotional and task-oriented).
- Most people become volunteers after being asked to volunteer by a friend, family member or a person known to them who is already volunteering. People are flattered when asked to volunteer even if they decline, although research tells us that 90 per cent of people who are directly invited to volunteer agree to do so.
- Finding male volunteers can be difficult. Recruitment campaigns should focus on what that volunteering activity could mean for the men who take it up. Organisations that work with children can provide valuable experience in parenting skills or as an area of future employment where men are under-represented. High schools, colleges and universities are possible sources for male volunteers. Service environments can be confusing to the newcomer so some direction as to the specific type of activity the male volunteer could take on – whether in the reading corner or on the playground – would help orient the newly recruited male volunteer (Wymer and Starness 2001; Ewing et al. 2002; Mejis and Hoogstad 2001).

CASE STUDY 4.3:   SURE START AND THE PAYMENT OF VOLUNTEERS

The issue of what remuneration, if any, volunteers should receive is not an easy one to get right, and each service organisation will have its own policies. Sure Start Blurton drew on the efforts of parent volunteers to undertake a large survey of parents who were using Sure Start Services. The scheme paid them for their time as they undertook the training for handling the questionnaire and for the interviewing. This raised the broader issue of whether parents who engage in other Sure Start activities should in some way receive recompense for their time and expertise. Because of the impact on individual benefit levels, however, no firm conclusions were taken on this. One idea is that voluntary activity could be broadened to include work parents carry out as board members or other similarly demanding roles such as participating in community forums. This would make them eligible for training grants with the possibility of securing tax credits for active citizenship.

BOX 4.2:   BASIC GUARANTEES FOR COMMUNITY REPRESENTATIVES WHO VOLUNTEER THEIR TIME

- Pay all out-of-pocket expenses, when the expense occurs or as soon as possible afterwards.
- Provide training/support for all board members, with some specifically targeted at community representatives.
- Meet at the most convenient time for all members.
- Give community representatives a chance to review their progress and contribution by linking them with staff, other board members or outsiders.
- Agree with the board a clear code of conduct that applies to all members.
- Pair mentors with new members to help them get into their role, perhaps with another board member or an outsider with relevant skills.
- Agree a personal development plan for each board member, tailored to their needs and aspirations.
- Carry out a skills audit to find out what added qualities people bring to the board.

KEY POINTS

☐   Citizen engagement includes the participation and empowerment of local people. Engagement is now essential for all services, as a result of a strong steer from central government but also from pressure by a better-informed public that wants to be involved in various ways.

☐ There are many barriers, however, to participation of the kind now expected of local people, especially for those living in disadvantaged neighbourhoods where expectations of services are low and previous experiences have taught people to remain suspicious of 'bogus empowerment'.

☐ There are a range of approaches that will promote public involvement, including community development, community learning and neighbourhood agreements. Practitioners should also pay close attention to the nuts and bolts of running good meetings, and of using different ways of drawing out local people's views on issues and concerns.

CHAPTER 5

NEIGHBOURHOOD SERVICES FOR CHILDREN AND FAMILIES

OBJECTIVES

By the end of this chapter you should:

- Understand the importance of neighbourhood environment in child development

- Be able to make connections between day-to-day practice and the outcomes for children in the government's *Every Child Matters* programme

- Be familiar with the common assessment framework as a key to unlocking responsive holistic services that take due account of environmental impacts and promote family competence in the locality

- Understand the importance of the early years and the critical role and skills of the early years professional

- Focus on schools as key hubs for children's services.

This chapter explores the contribution of neighbourhood-based services to enhancing children's well-being and promoting stronger families. It begins by looking at the importance of neighbourhood in children's development, and introduces the 'ecological theory' as a way of incorporating elements of a child's environment in our overall understanding of a particular child and children in general. The chapter then moves to ways of assessing the impact of environment on children's lives and behaviour, by giving greater prominence to neighbourhood influences within the assessment framework. The chapter finally looks at kinds of community-based and community-level services that are being developed for children and parents, particularly those using schools as hubs for delivery.

The state of childhood and the kind of life children now lead has become a pressing national issue. Parents, the public, government policy makers and professionals from many disciplines are all voicing concerns about the pressures and stresses facing children and young people. The big questions, once the preserve of psychologists teachers and social workers, have moved into the public domain. Do parents know enough about parenting or should they be taught? At what age should children attend play and education centres or day care? For how long? Why is there a huge rise in rates of autistic spectrum disorders and behavioural disorders? What effect does separation and divorce have on children? Are we protecting our children too much? Or not enough? Are they falling behind in literacy and maths? Or do we over-test them? What is happening to childhood itself? Is there time enough for play, exploration of interests and hobbies, cycling and pick-up games of jump rope or cricket?

All of the above are critical issues with no easy answers to hand. But what is important for practitioners to realise is that now the public as a whole and certainly parents are closely involved in their quest for answers: gathering information, testing their perspectives, needing discussion and expecting to be heard. They are doing so out of necessity. They want ideas and information on what is the right balance between work and raising and loving their children. Many parents believe that the contemporary conditions of childhood contrast unfavourably to their own, that Britain has become a less child-friendly nation and that they, the parents, have to fight for the kind of life they want for their children – with no guarantee of success. They sense that consumerism is 'infiltrating the intimate relationship of child and parent and subtly undermining parental authority' as Madeleine Bunting has put it (Bunting 2006a) and want to know how to stop it. But neither will they deferentially follow learned advice without question. They want to be involved in reaching answers, to develop their own information flows, to be consulted, to learn from and to teach others. In short, the old presumption of deference to experts on childhood no longer works because it is clear to all that the issues are too large and too deep and that no one, professionals included, has sufficient answers.

Neighbourhood-centred services are based on the realisation that problems for children, families and communities are strongly interlinked. When viewed as a continuum such services are a seamless way of distributing practitioners' activities and commitments across a wide spectrum of family realities that reflect particular strengths and weaknesses and resilience and risks of those families over time (Mulroy *et al.* 2005). Strong direct practice skills are needed as well as the capacity to work in informal settings, whether rooms in community centres, church halls, or a room booked in a clinic or youth centre. Practitioners need to be able to work across organisational boundaries in order to create new programmes.

THE IMPORTANCE OF NEIGHBOURHOOD ENVIRONMENTS IN CHILDREN'S DEVELOPMENT

The more we understand of children's development, the more clearly we see the connection between a child's well-being and that of their family and neighbourhood around them. These influences may be *direct*, such as a neighbourhood characterised by structural dimensions such as income (whether high or low) and poor services, or *indirect* through their impact on family functioning and parental behaviour. Parents act as brokers and advocates for their children in obtaining neighbourhood resources – whether tangible assets such as play space or good primary schools or intangible assets such as community safety. But these roles are now circumscribed. For example, the loss of play areas and particularly street space for children's games has been swift and unremitting. Using 'the street' as an emblem for all outdoor spaces in public, its loss represents a severe rupture in opportunities for parents to make safe play arrangements (Barnes *et al.* 2006).

The level of these resources in any given neighbourhood is critical to what parents can obtain for their children. Leventhal and Brooks-Gunn (2000) examined the pathways through which neighbourhood effects are transmitted to children and young people. They identified:

1   Institutional resources: the availability, accessibility, affordability and quality of learning, social and recreational activities, child care, schools and medical facilities.
2   Relationships: parental characteristics (such as mental health including level of irritability, coping skills, and physical health), extent of support networks, parental behaviour including warmth, degrees of harshness and control, and the home environment. These parental relationships in effect mediate neighbourhood characteristics in relation to their children's well-being.
3   Norms and collective efficacy: the extent to which community-level institutions and informal controls exist in the neighbourhood to supervise and monitor the behaviour of residents (including young people's behaviour) and the extent of physical risk through victimisation, violence or drug usage.

A local children's service requires mapping neighbourhood resources and looking at them in light of the role they play in shaping the child–parent relationship. The resources include:

•   the quality of services such as playgroups and pre-school centres, schools, housing
•   the geography of safety and risk – the particular streets, shops, high-rise foyers or play areas where children know themselves to be safe or in jeopardy
•   the employment or training opportunities for parents and level of parental income
•   the strengths and stresses found within the social networks and associational life of the neighbourhood – for example the level of volunteering, vibrancy of local institutions and the degree of 'efficacy' and trust.

Practitioners should not assume that children and parents living in disadvantaged neighbourhoods automatically have a negative opinion of their environment. Seaman *et al.* (2006) have recently reported a cluster of findings that bear directly on our perception of how services should be constructed within localities. They concluded that how parents and young people engaged with their communities provided an important element of their resilience and in keeping them safe. They found for instance that, despite the lived experience of deprivation within their localities – poverty, unemployment, organised gangs, drug addiction – parents and young people found positive aspects about living in their local areas such as the presence of trusted family friends and neighbours. Far from being victimised by the range of multiple and overlapping deprivations existing within the neighbourhood, both parents and children had adopted strategies and tactics for coping with the local risks and maximising their well-being. Parents did not emerge in this study as ill-informed, ineffectual disciplinarians who required sharp lessons in child management. Rather, they employed open parenting styles that were democratic and sophisticated, and worked alongside their children to keep them safe.

The ecological model

The ecological model is now widely recognised as a way of understanding and representing how the different elements of the child's world relate one to another. Developed by the social psychologist Uri Bronfenbrenner (Bronfenbrenner 1979), it lays out the relationship between a child and her or his environment in a series of layers, often represented as concentric circles. The inner circle immediately surrounding the child is the *micro system* – in which the child develops relationships with those closest to her or him such as parents, relatives and siblings. The *meso system* includes both the immediate family and the pre-school, playgroup or school that the child attends as well as any other association or joining activity the child attends regularly. The *exo system* is more removed from the child but nevertheless exerts powerful effects on the child's life: for example the parents's workplace, with its capacity to absorb parental time (or render the parent unemployed), volunteer activity and other attributes of the civil society in which the child is being raised, but could also include more directly malign associations – obtaining drugs or alcohol. Finally there is the *macro system* – the overarching structure of society in which the legal framework and economic activity are foremost.

The way in which the model is portrayed in four concentric circles is misleading. It seems to suggest that each of the different levels are self-contained and that there is a practice competence related to each but not one that extends across all four. In fact the ecological model is a construction of the way a child's life unfolds: in that life course all factors are intertwined and are having an impact all the time on the child. Consequently practitioners' competences needs to engage at all levels.

The ecological model is not deterministic: through these four systems the child develops and makes his or her way through choices of their own and of their parents. What the child and its parents encounter are seen by them as life events – they remain goal directed, wanting to achieve meaning and a sense of well-being (Briggs 2002). What the model achieves is to illuminate the different levels of a child's developmental environment in which these choices are made, and points out that to reach a flourishing young adulthood well-being is more than a linear progression of a life unfolding. As Utting *et al.* have put it (2002: 12), 'children's wellbeing amounts to more than the successful completion of developmental tasks at different ages and states. Children's wellbeing, or their wellness, is determined by the level of family and community wellbeing.'

The contemporary significance of the ecological model cannot be overstated. It has provided a major starting point for understanding the link between children and their community, and specifically the realisation that simply looking at the child in terms of developmental stages or as confined only to a family system is insufficient for

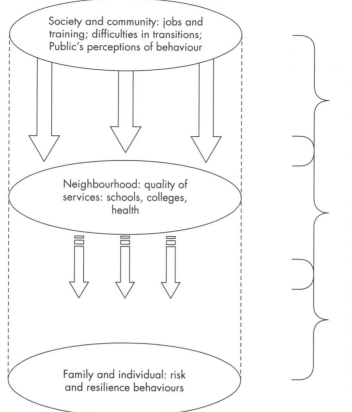

FIGURE 5.1 The ecological model: children and young people shaped by their wider environment

assessing and understanding that child's behaviour (Jack and Jack 2000). As Department of Health guidance has put it, 'Whilst the significance of understanding the parent/child relationship has long been part of social services' practice, the importance has not always been recognised of the interface between environmental considerations and a child's development and the influence of environmental factors on parents' capacity to respond to the child's needs' (DoH 2000: 11).

The ecological model is not without limitations. It is a system-based theory, which, in Houston's phrase, 'generally tends to overplay societal consensus, stability and integration' (Houston 2002: 304). While poverty is rightly highlighted as an impediment to cohesive social networks, it lacks 'a firm grounding in political economy [and] ends up as an inert category' (Houston 2002: 304). This limitation goes some way to explaining how social work simply incorporated the Department of Health's Framework for Assessment of Children in Need (DoH 2000) into its existing assessment practice but did not really take seriously what Jack and Gill (2003) call 'the missing side of the triangle' – that is identifying the strengths and weaknesses in the child's community and environment and planning interventions accordingly.

OUTCOMES AND *EVERY CHILD MATTERS*

The publication of *Every Child Matters* (DfES 2003), the government's promotion of its related agenda for change and the Children Act 2004 push practitioners beyond the scope of the Framework for Assessment into a direct encounter with outcomes for children. The overhaul of services includes the formation of children's trusts, locating children's services within the Department for Education and Skills and committing all practitioners to intervention in neighbourhood environments.

The five outcomes for children

Every Child Matters lays out five outcomes that practitioners from whatever service or organisation, public or voluntary, must promote in relation to the children they work with. (This is in contrast with seven 'life dimensions' of the *Assessment Framework* (DoH, 2000).) As we noted in Chapter two, the concept of outcomes is dynamic – pressing practitioners to look at children in terms of aspects of their well-being and to deliver services accordingly. The five outcomes for children are:

- being healthy: enjoying good physical and mental health and living a healthy lifestyle
- staying safe: being protected from harm and neglect
- enjoying and achieving: getting the most out of life and developing the skills for adulthood
- making a positive contribution: being involved with the community and society and not engaging in anti-social or offending behaviour
- achieving economic well-being: *not* being prevented by economic disadvantage from achieving their full potential (DfES 2003).

These outcomes are not to be confused with outputs that attempt to measure the take-up of a service (Axford and Berry 2005). The number of children taking part in a homework club after school or in a 'stay and play' Sure Start scheme for parents or who are being fostered in a given area is an output, not an outcome. The *Every Child Matters* programme attempts to capture whether children enjoy improved levels of well-being regardless of what service system they are in contact with, for example school, youth justice, health and sexual health promotion. If they enjoy good physical health, are safe from abuse and exploitation and show better behavioural and cognitive development than they would have otherwise enjoyed had they or their families not received the services, then children's services will have done what they are supposed to do. Axford and Berry define outcomes this way: 'A useful rule of thumb is that the things that we are concerned with for our own children invariably relate to outcomes not outputs' (2005: 13).

ACTIVITY 5.1: THE DIFFICULTIES IN FOCUSING ON OUTCOMES

The notion of outcomes can seem distant, overly general and out of reach to practitioners in their day-to-day work as they struggle to achieve agency targets. Think of the outcomes government has laid down in *Every Child Matters*. What progress has your agency made towards them? What factors, obstacles or ways of thinking make such outcomes difficult to achieve?

Creating the outcome culture in a multi-disciplinary context

Only strong local partnerships in which the local authorities work with other partners to assess local needs and commission services to meet them will bring about the needed changes to frontline services to deliver outcomes. Increasingly children's trusts bring together public, private, voluntary and community organisations to work together to shape the children's services in their particular area: primary care trusts, local authorities, police, schools, voluntary and community organisations, and children, young people and families. Uniting locally delivered services around outcomes is not always smooth. Tensions, particularly around resource allocations, arise between those parts of the service focused on risk and safeguarding children and those arms of the service focusing on prevention, building resilience in children and in particular those attempting to deliver community-level services (Axford and Berry 2005: 12).

BOX 5.1   THE CHILDREN ACT 2004

Every Child Matters emphasises multi-disciplinary and community-based provision as part of a strategy to tackle fragmentation and long-standing lack of accountability in children's services. The Children Act 2004 pursues this by requiring in each area an integrated strategy of joint assessments of local needs of children, young people and their parents, and the delivery of integrated frontline services to improve outcomes for children. It:

- creates a Children's Commissioner to champion the views and interests of children and young people
- places a duty on local authorities to make arrangements to promote cooperation between agencies and other appropriate bodies in order to improve children's well-being and places a duty on key partners, including primary care trusts and NHS trusts, to take part in these collaborative arrangements
- places a duty on all key agencies to safeguard and promote the welfare of children and for the local authority to set up a board to oversee the safeguarding of children

- includes provision for databases containing basic information about children and young people to enable better sharing of information
- lays down a requirement for a single children and young people's plan to be drawn up by each local authority
- includes a requirement for local authorities to appoint a director of children's services and to designate a lead member from the local council
- requires the creation of an integrated inspection framework and the conduct of Joint Area Reviews to assess local areas' progress in improving outcomes and in provisions relating to foster care, private fostering and the education of children in care.

LINKING COMMUNITY BUILDING WITH SERVICES FOR CHILDREN

As the impact of neighbourhood and community environments on children's lives has become clearer, so has the realisation that for children's services to be effective they have to engage more directly with that environment. Since the mid 1990s this work has moved forward in the UK, the US, Canada and Australia. Family centres, community development and regeneration initiatives (Cannan and Warren 1997), anti-poverty programmes and neighbourhood-based early years programmes such as Sure Start in the UK or Early Head Start in the US have all focused on the link between improving child outcomes and building effective capacity in disadvantaged neighbourhoods.

Some initiatives are aimed at community level. The target for change is the neighbourhood or community itself through which local people develop the skills and capacities to solve problems, change behaviour and exert informal controls. Others are community based, that is intending to support specific families in improving the outcomes for their children (Barnes *et al*. 2006). Sure Start, the early years neighbourhood-based programme in the UK, is a good example of both kinds of services. It sought to raise the understanding of entire neighbourhoods in relation to warm and nurturing parenting styles, the benefits of breastfeeding, the risks to the child of drinking and smoking during pregnancy. It also provided individual families with support through locally based baby clinics, increased health visitor involvement, speech and language advice, and psychological services for post-natal depression.

The overall goal is what might broadly be called a 'healthy community' in which children can flourish. Such a community would embrace economic and physical security, environmental and public safety, nurturing and stable family environments, adult role models and mentors, positive peer activities, and decent schools and health care (Mulroy *et al*. 2005).

Mulroy and her colleagues identify three elements that should be present in order to at least make some progress toward this ambitious aim:

- strong community-based organisations, often local voluntary organisations, that can offer programmes and means for participation that meet residents' needs
- a full spectrum of services that tackle disadvantage, build capacity, offer informal support and provide early intervention as well as formal interventions such as family group conferencing and safeguarding children
- close interagency collaboration (Mulroy *et al*. 2005).

The skills for what might be called the 'community building' approach to children's services draw on much of what social workers already do: they need to be able to create constructive relationships, work across organisational boundaries, manage information, help facilitate groups, launch a range of informal community contacts, and nurture the strengths and talents of local people.

The remainder of this chapter provides different ways of how to achieve the outcomes of *Every Child Matters* through the community building approach.

ASSESSMENT OF CHILDREN AND FAMILIES: PAYING CLOSE ATTENTION TO 'THE MISSING SIDE OF THE TRIANGLE'

Experienced practitioners will be familiar with the framework for assessment of children in need which the Department of Health developed in 2000. It asks all those involved in assessing a child in need to consider three domains of a child's life: i) the child's developmental needs including emotional and behavioural development, ii) the parents capacity to provide basic care, emotional warmth and stimulation and iii) family and environmental factors. Within the framework, presented as three sides of a triangle, theories of attachment and child development merged with heightened focus on the child's environment and in particular drew on ecological theory to integrate these three domains.

Historically social work has felt its natural competence to fall only on the individual and familial sides, leaving a gap in relation to how that third domain, which includes community resources, family social networks, parents' income and employment and housing, more closely shapes children's lives. But the development of holistic neighbourhood services points strongly to understanding more specifically the impact of neighbourhood and community environment on children in need.

Jack and Gill have produced a useful model for analysing this 'missing side of the triangle' (2003). Their approach, based on the ecological model, highlights key areas of information as part of the assessment process that social workers often down play or ignore altogether (see Figure 5.2). These include:

- The interaction between a family and available community resources, and the factors that may be limiting their use of those resources. This requires practitioners to look not only at internal family dynamics but also at the level of local resources such as child care and their accessibility. It also requires practitioners to become familiar with the range of informal services such as local play facilities, open access youth centres and what Jack and Gill define as 'home zones', where one or more residential streets are subject to vastly reduced traffic with the introduction of trees, seating and environmental changes that make that part of the neighbourhood pedestrian focused and convivial in nature (Jack and Gill 2003: 25).
- The extent of the child's social integration in terms of local relationships and the degree to which the child has been able to develop significant relationships outside the family. Such relationships begin in pre-school and as the child grows become more important in relation to school and neighbourhood peer groups. Their degree of supportiveness or rejection plays an important role in the child's emerging

identity and behaviour. But in determining this the practitioner must bear in mind that housing location, income level and family finances, and parental employment all shape the way a child and its family are able to find inclusion or not in a given area.

The point here is not to make practitioners feel responsible for all elements of the third side of the assessment triangle but first to begin the task of rebalancing their work towards assessing more fully the extent of community stressors faced by individual families, and second to concentrate on minimising one or two of the environmental pressures as directly relevant to work with the family. It is also to plan, in conjunction with others, how joint action might promote a child's well-being by tackling these stressors.

Mapping the neighbourhood from children's point of view

Children themselves know their own locality more intimately than adults. Rasmussen and Smidt drew on children's photo journals to help them pin down the very physical way in which children view their neighbourhoods. Children between the ages of 5 and 12 were asked to photograph the places they visited and the activities they were involved in, which Rasmussen and Smidt then categorised. These categories included:

- places used such as playgrounds, earth mounds to dig in, shacks, dens, swings in trees
- means of transport such as bicycles, home-made go-carts, parents' car and roller blades
- nature spots such as trees, stone walls, small gardens
- public buildings and places such as water towers, building sites, corner shops, shopping centres, sports centres, bus shelters, structures at recreation grounds
- private buildings and places such as family homes and gardens
- special persons with a connection to the neighbourhood such as shopkeeper or friends (Rasmussen and Smidt 2003 cited in Barnes *et al.* 2006).

The common assessment framework

The common assessment framework (CAF) is a single, combined assessment process shared by all elements of children's services for those children who may be in need. It encourages a move away from exclusive focus on short-term targets to develop a longer-term view of how services should be deployed across the whole life of the child. It presses these services to identify how the absence of a particular service – for example support for parents on managing their child's behaviour or pre-school care and education – can lead to difficult, more costly problems later on.

The CAF strives to find a language and format that all agencies can use to assess the complex interaction between children's development and their environment and how to decide when services should intervene to improve outcomes. The need for the CAF arose from the realisation that earlier arrangements for identifying and responding

STRENGTHS		PRESSURES	
PARENTS	**CHILDREN**	**PARENTS**	**CHILDREN**
1. Practical resources in the community			
Employment (links to income and social integration)	Anti-poverty resources (e.g. breakfast clubs, subsidised holidays)	High local levels of unemployment	Leisure facilities, outings and holidays are not affordable or accessible
Good local shops (for good quality, good value food)	Good quality, accessible play resources	Transport expensive, infrequent, unreliable	Lack of safe, local play areas/facilities
Transport (access to employment, friends and family, leisure); Credit unions, benefits advice	Specific resources for black, minority ethnic and disabled children	No access to financial advice or services	Few organised clubs and out of school activities
Social network developments (drop-in groups, community centres and community activities)	Social network development (e.g. after school clubs and playgroups)	Expensive credit facilities	No specific resources for black, minority ethnic children or children with disabilities
Affordable local child care and education (for children's development and parents' employment)	Local schools provide inclusive and supportive environment	Resources for child care and pre-school care and education are inadequate (number of places, opening hours, location, cost, level of staff training)	Local schools provide poor educational and social environments (e.g. low achievement, bullying, disruptive behaviour)
2. Natural networks in the community			
Reciprocal 'helping' relationships in community and neighbourhood	Established and supportive social networks	Culture of people 'keeping themselves to themselves'; social norms not enforced	Lack of positive contact with range of people in community
Long-term residence of families	Good contact with immediate neighbours	High rates of mobility in and out	Children's networks disrupted
Non-threatening relations with immediate neighbours	Positive contact with significant adults from different generations	Lack of links between wider family and community networks	Lack of links between school and community networks
3. Child and family safety in the community			
Community members perceived as safe (people safety)	Children perceive their immediate area to be safe, rather than threatening	Parents see community as unsafe (crime/drugs, lack of physical safety)	Children perceive local environment as threatening (people, crime/drugs, danger)

Community activities seen as safe		Harassment from neighbours	Harassment from adults and children
4. Community norms around children and child care			
Established positive community norms around childcare practice and values	Children experience stable and established community norms	Lack of established positive community norms around childcare practice and values	Children do not experience stable and established community norms
	Positive sense of identity and belonging conveyed to children	Teenagers, disabled, poor or minority ethnic children are isolated	Negative sense of identity conveyed to certain children
5. The individual family and child in the community			
Personal resources and knowledge to access available facilities	Developing confidence in using available facilities	Lack of personal resources or knowledge to access facilities	Lack of personal resources to access available facilities
Personal resources to develop and maintain supportive networks	Developing confidence in local networks with other children	Personal demands too high to develop reciprocal relationships	Alienates other children/other children bully or stigmatise
Perceptions that local facilities are accessible for their family	Perception that facilities are accessible to all including minority ethnic and disabled children	Alienates potential sources of support; Networks produce demands rather than support	Family networks either limited or difficult; Child has frequent moves (including homelessness)
6. Cumulative impact of all of the above			
Low level of individual environmental stress	Children feel their community is a good place to be living	High level of individual 'environmental stress' (poor housing, lack of childcare)	Children feel threatened, frightened and unvalued in their community
Feel supported in the community in their parental role of brining up children	Children feel safe and valued in their community	Parents feel unsupported, threatened or frightened in their community	Anxiety, depression, anti-social behaviour, school failure/exclusion
Community/neighbourhood is perceived as a 'good place to bring up children'	Development of positive identity, self-esteem and security	Parents' ambitions are to leave the community	

FIGURE 5.2 Jack and Gill's model of stresses and pressures

to the needs of children were not sufficiently outcome based. This earlier culture of assessment tended to assess particular aspects of a child's welfare while overlooking other dimensions and needs. It also tended to ignore previous assessments of the child. But perhaps the biggest fault of the old approach was to use it simply as a way of making a decision as to whether a child met or did not meet the threshold for a service offered by the assessing agency (DfES 2004). In short the assessment objectives were about outputs (whether or not a child qualified for a particular service) and not about outcomes (the child's well-being). The CAF's purpose is expressly to move away from an assessment culture dominated by the statutory obligations of particular services (DfEs 2004).

The CAF then is intended for use when there is an early sign of difficulty in a child's life, to identify further supports should these be needed. The assessment takes place within a universal setting such as nursery or primary school or a care and education pre-school. A multi-agency approach is likely to be required so that information can be shared between agencies. It is intended as a 'front end' to the assessment process, a mechanism through which any practitioner working with a child or young person can conduct a good-quality, but relatively non-specialised, assessment. Above all, parents and children where at all possible should be involved in it and be able to understand the process at every step. It is specifically non-bureaucratic and looks at the whole child in the ecological sense. Should a more specialised service be required, the CAF helps ensure that the referral is made.

BOX 5.2: COMMON ASSESSMENT FRAMEWORK

The common assessment framework (CAF) should provide:

- a common set of processes for practitioners to follow if they think a child or young person would benefit from a common assessment
- a common method for assessing the needs of children and young people based on models of successful children's development and concepts of well-being
- supporting guidance to help practitioners record their findings, including gaining appropriate consent
- requirements and guidance as to the roles and responsibilities of agencies and practitioners.

The CAF developed locally should reflect local patterns of service delivery and priorities. Particularly significant is the size of the network to be trained in using the CAF. DfES guidance makes it clear that *all* practitioners in an area who provide services for children should know about the CAF and how to complete it.

The reach of the CAF is wider than the assessment framework for children in need. It is triggered when a practitioner from any setting judges that a child or young person may have additional needs which are not then being met but which have to be met if the child is to achieve his or her potential in relation to the five outcomes of *Every Child Matters*.

(adapted from *Common Assessment Framework Consultation*, DfES 2004)

THE IMPORTANCE OF THE EARLY YEARS IN ACHIEVING SUCCESSFUL OUTCOMES

Early attachments, environmental circumstances and parenting styles – authoritative, rather than authoritarian or permissive – heavily impact early brain development. Over the last fifteen years a wealth of research has reported how this happens. Neurological research for example has shown how responsive to environment an infant's brain is.

Thus neither 'nurture' nor 'nature' are influential in their own right but actually cannot be defined concretely without relationship to the other (Shonkoff and Phillips 2001). Shonkoff and Phillips describe the interrelationship between environment and a child's natural endowments as one of 'coactivity' (Shonkoff and Phillips 2001: 41). They write:

> Hereditary vulnerability establishes . . . developmental pathways that evolve in concert with experiential stressors, or buffers, in the family, the neighbourhood and the school. That is why early experiences of abuse, neglect, poverty, and family violence are of such concern. They are likely to enlist the genetic vulnerabilities of some children into a downward spiral of progressive dysfunction.
>
> (Shonkoff and Phillips 2001: 55–6)

Recent studies of anti-social behaviour in adopted children found that 'when biological parents had substance abuse problems or antisocial personality disorder their adopted children were much more likely to be hostile and antisocial than were adoptees from untroubled biological parents' (Shonkoff and Phillips 2001: 42). The practical implication of this is that environmental influences can moderate the development of inherited tendencies, making the construction of a supportive context worthwhile. These contexts must vary: rambunctious children need opportunities for exuberance and physical activity while shy children need places of retreat. It is important that families and service providers understand the necessary fit between inherited vulnerabilities and behavioural demands, especially for ADHD, depression and anti-social behaviour (Shonkoff and Phillips 2001).

In the first two years of life the child passes through a number of thresholds that mark moving from individually mediated learning to wider socially based learning. For example, paying attention as part of a group, participating in social routines, responding with feeling to reciprocally developing relationships, engaging in independent, purposeful and sustained activities and use of language to establish joint meanings are all indicators of this development.

BOX 5.3: THE CHILDCARE ACT 2006

The overriding importance of the early years for children's development is now enshrined in law with the passage of the Childcare Act 2006, which makes accessible high-quality child care and services for children under five for all families. It is intended to put early childhood

continued

services in the mainstream of local authority activity – and thereby to signal to parents, whatever their background, that services developed first within the Sure Start local programmes will continue within the framework of children centres.

It does this by assigning new statutory duties to local authorities to:

- improve the outcomes of all children under five and close the gap between children in areas of the poorest outcomes and the rest through early childhood services that are integrated, proactive and readily available
- develop the child care market in their area to ensure that it meets the needs of working parents, especially those on low incomes and with disabled children
- introduce the Early Years Foundation Stage which integrates education and care for children from birth to five
- focus on raising the quality of the pre-school care and education by reducing the regulatory framework.

The Childcare Act 2006 also lays a duty on top-tier local authorities to improve the five outcomes from *Every Child Matters* for all under fives in their area. The integrated services must embrace early education and child care, social services, relevant health services (health visitors, ante-natal and post-natal care), information services and Jobcentre Plus to help parents obtain work. The act further underscores the way early years services are to be delivered: integrated provision in order to facilitate access and optimise benefits to users; outreach to ensure that those families needing services are identified and engaged, including fathers; involvement of parents – fathers and mothers – in service planning and delivery as well as providers from the private and voluntary sectors.

Parental support

We know that the relationships within families and the quality of parenting are more important to children's development than specific family structures. We are also clearer on what works in parenting support:

- the processes of service provision – the relationships developed, the attitudes of practitioners and *how* programmes are delivered – are more important than content
- in any locality there should be a range of universal, open-access services as well as targeted services with staff appropriately trained for each
- engage parents and children together, particularly when children are young
- continuous outreach to parents is essential to keep parents engaged in a programme
- parents learn well from sharing experiences with other parents (but need individual work when problems are entrenched)
- for many parents the level of stress or economic factors are the highest priority and must be addressed first (Moran *et al.* 2004).

Parents themselves are looking for services that:

- are timely and accessible and there when needed
- meet parents' own self-defined needs
- are informative
- respect their expertise in relation to their own lives
- regard highly their sense of responsibility and do not undermine their own sense of autonomy (Ghate and Hazel 2002).

We know also that they most readily turn to health visitors, GPs or their own parents when in need of advice (Gill *et al.* 2002).

Government has gone a considerable way to lay the foundation for a child- and family-centred provision in each locality, particularly for children under five where historically provision has been scant. This includes the formation of Sure Start children's centres in disadvantaged areas and the development of children's centres in every community by 2010. Services at the centres include pre-school care and education that will follow the government-mandated foundation curriculum year by year from birth to five. The centres will also provide information and advice including ante-natal and post natal health advice and speech and language development services. Following the national evaluation of Sure Start local programmes, a more determined effort is under way to keep 'hard to reach' families within service tracks through home visiting and a growing spread of voluntary and peer outreach programmes such as PIPPIN, and Strengthening Families, Strengthening Communities (Barnes *et al.* 2006).

Tackling low socio-economic neighbourhood environments

There is however considerable space in which child-dedicated practitioners can and must innovate, particularly in ensuring that families receive the resources they need. The single most important research finding of the last ten years relating to children is Leon Feinstein's investigation into the role that inequality plays in shaping children's cognitive development (Feinstein 2003; Feinstein 2007). Broadly his research demonstrates that children with good cognitive skills but born into families and areas dominated by disadvantage and low socio-economic status *lose* those skills because the environment does not support them. Thus children with high cognitive skills at 22 months but living in low status socio-economic environments have largely lost those skills by age seven. On the other hand children with low cognitive skills at 22 months but born into high socio-economic environments have steadily improved on their attainments. By age 10 the apparent cognitive abilities of the two groups have been reversed.

Feinstein makes a further point. The same damaging impact of social and economic background on cognitive ability rolls on through childhood but does not follow a linear path. It is not the case that at age five (or seven) the damage is final; high achieving seven year olds continue to be damaged by disadvantaged backgrounds as do high achieving 11 year olds. The cause is the same: *low social and economic status in time overcomes the resilience of children* (Feinstein, 2007); and the conclusion is the same: *children know when they are at the disadvantaged end of the unequal society they live in – they know it and they suffer as a result.*

A number of leads open out from Feinstein's work. One is the vital role that practitioners play at local level in directing resources, advocating for families, and attacking child poverty. Their local knowledge, Feinstein argues, is essential in figuring out how to link income, work opportunities and child care options for families who need it most. A second lead arises from practitioners' intermediary position within service delivery partnerships: they can see the connections between i) family factors such as size, income and level of poverty ii) characteristics of the family such as physical and mental health of parents or parents' cognitive attainments and iii) parenting advice and capacity for home learning (Feinstein 2007). From this vantage point a skilled determination as to how resources should be deployed becomes possible. A third lead is the bending of integrated services to tackle the effects of low socio-economic environments whether working closely with schools, on for example pupil selection policies, or with the police in burglary reduction and domestic abuse initiatives, or with local employers in job provision.

BOX 5.4: THE CASE FOR EARLY YEARS PROGRAMMES ON GROUNDS OF COSTS

Early years services have been found to be highly efficient for public investment. This is because such services reduce the expenditure on corrective and remediation services later in a child or young person's life. These savings are found in four broad areas: lower costs for education services, reduction in welfare costs, reduction in criminal justice costs and increased taxes from higher levels of employment.

In the area of criminal justice, for example, are the costs of youth offending later in the life cycle of children who by early adolescence have fallen into a pattern of anti-social and criminal behaviour. There are costs for those individuals who have failed to develop sufficient skills to allow them to participate in the labour market as young adults with a resulting loss of taxes to the exchequer *and* the additional welfare costs associated with non-participation in the labour market. The costs of remedial education are incurred earlier in the child's life, for example in the form of one-on-one classroom support for those with special needs or other services, whether defined by a statement from the local authority or, as is more commonly the case, left to the individual school to devise an informal support package

(Carneiro and Heckman 2003: 89).

WORKING WITH AND THROUGH SCHOOLS

Researchers have long recognised that changing parental behaviour in ways that enhances the well-being of the child is often difficult. The paradox is that despite parental influence predominating in shaping outcomes, improvements to child outcomes are more easily secured in care and education settings, after the age of three (Waldfogel 2005).

As a result schools have become important settings in the locality for achieving the five outcomes of *Every Child Matters*. While schools have long been recognised as places for improving the health and emotional well-being of children through school dinners, milk, vaccinations and counselling, only since the Children Act 2004 has children's policy formally brought education and children's social services together.

BOX 5.5: WHAT PRIMARY SCHOOL CHILDREN LOOK FOR IN THEIR SCHOOL

Primary pupils are particularly concerned about the quality of their relationships, and mentioned friendship and loneliness and what needs to be done to enrich social relationships. Knowing that there would be supportive adults around was as important as having special people (including trained peers) to provide assistance. Said one primary pupil:

> When, like, someone is lonely, they [adults in school] help them . . . if they've got a problem. . . . It makes people feel happier instead of them being on their own. . . . If you get shouted at all the time it makes you feel bad inside, but if you get nice people and get on well with them then you feel good inside

(Warwick *et al.* 2005).

The advantages of working through schools are many. They provide both universal and targeted services, a multi-agency platform for joined up services, and legitimacy in the locality. National Healthy Schools Standards, sexual health, Health Action Zones, drug awareness programmes, and citizenship education all focus on elements of the child's environment and seek to provide the child with the information and sense of role, responsibility and potential that allows them to take their rightful place within that environment. It is increasingly recognised that services offered through schools happen in a non-stigmatising environment.

There is also evidence that schools provide a ready channel for working with parents and 'whole family' involvement – helping parents manage difficult behaviour and boosting their knowledge of child development. As local institutions with wide legitimacy schools can also offer a holistic approach. As Pugh and Statham put it:

> A whole school approach which improves the emotional climate of the school and builds on relationships with families, is more likely to promote the well-being of all children *and to form a sound basis for more structured and sustained intervention for those children with particular needs* (my italics).

(Pugh and Stratham 2006: 288)

What Pugh and Statham have in mind are school-based interventions that enhance children's well-being by:

- increasing self-esteem, self-awareness and self-confidence
- promoting attachment and developmental catch up
- improving relationships and peer acceptance

- improving educational attainment
- bringing attention to bear on the needs of vulnerable children.

One of the ways of achieving these is through home–school link projects. They cover a fast proliferating cluster of service activity – providing home visits, parental support with children who engage in difficult behaviour, anti-bullying, mentoring, befriending and other forms of peer support. Promoting positive mental health is a thread common to many such programmes as they respond to complex links between rising mental health problems in children, problematic child behaviour and school exclusions. Nurture groups in primary schools, after-school clubs and homework clubs all feature in the extended school model (Boxall 2002).

Social worker relationships with schools have been partial and at times not easy. For a profession like social work, whose culture is wedded to the notions of the uniqueness of individuals and individual autonomy, the hierarchical and rule-based school system can at times seem inherently antagonistic to working with troubled young people. To a certain extent the policy and practice outlined in the schools white paper of 2005 potentially aggravates this relationship further since it makes pupil selection and local autonomy for schools a priority (DfES 2005a). Schools can become self-governing trusts, independent of local authorities, and set their own admissions policies. In selecting pupils this may lead to an emphasis on parental background, pupil potential for high test scores and, indirectly, weight admissions against children from low-income families and vulnerable children. Children's services on the other hand are counting on schools to play a key role in delivering the outcomes of *Every Child Matters*. This leaves the practitioner in a difficult position that requires brokering, collaborative and negotiation skills able to hold schools to account on behalf of children and their communities, particularly with regard to the admission or exclusion of particular pupils.

CASE STUDY 5.1: EDUCATION PARTNERSHIP AND BLACON EDUCATIONAL VILLAGE

An audit of educational provision and problems within the Blacon estate near Chester has revealed some key issues. The number of children in the community has been falling for some time and there is no sign of an upturn in the birthrate in the near future. These pupil demographics have had consequences for schools' finances in that falling numbers have led to the withdrawal of funding for core teaching and support posts. These realities, together with persistent concerns about local people's perception of Blacon schools, has led to all stakeholders concluding that they need to work together rather than competing. Cooperative relationships between schools have been predicated upon a negotiated shared vision of the children's and the community's needs, and this has subsequently led to shared policies and to more rational decisions being made about the use of scarce resources. The policies have included matters concerning bullying, dealing with racism, promoting and valuing diversity, drugs training and early years provision (the latter is perceived as key in relation to the government's overall child care strategy – currently under review again).

The community plays a close and supportive role in the partnership. It:

- provides volunteer observers to report on truancy, positive activities of families and children and home/school watch
- offers skills and resources available such as entrepreneurship and business skills, retired people's skills in organisation and management, mentoring and support for children and young people, as well as filling civic roles such as school governorships
- acts as an advocate for schools and disseminates good practice and positive achievements
- challenges parents' condoned absences and tries to influence (positively) hard to reach families/ parents.

In relation to the question 'what might schools do for the community?' the key suggestions are to:

- promote inter-school activities so that schools can enjoy each other's facilities/advantages
- encourage the use of school facilities/premises/grounds by the community
- become more involved in the local festival
- provide open days for the community to become involved in policies and have them explained
- publicise the achievements of children and schools in 'one voice'.

Family learning

The link between parenting and schools is critical to the educational progress of children. Parental involvement in their child's school has long provided one indicator as to how well that child will do in school but also across other domains such as behaviour and achievement in early adulthood (DfES 2003).

One way to consolidate parental involvement is through family learning projects. Through these parents are invited into schools – although sometimes they are held in libraries and community centres – to work alongside their children and to learn what they are being taught and how. Programmes can vary in that parents may in fact concentrate more on their own learning – such as literacy or numeracy. They are particularly positive in areas where there are new arrivals to Britain or minority ethnic communities, providing the opportunity to improve English skills as well as making social contact (London West Learning and Skills Council 2005).

CASE STUDY 5.2: SCHOOL HOME SUPPORT

Lewisham's vulnerable young children's team aims to increase the social inclusion of children and families and to work with schools to reduce students' emotional and behavioural difficulties.

continued

It draws on School Home Support, an independent agency that works with children and families at school, and the child and adolescent mental health services team, itself located with Lewisham's behavioural education support team. The team works with children at school because that is where they mostly are and in surroundings they are familiar with. It puts a School Home Support worker in five primary schools, and a designated children and adolescent mental health (CAMHS) worker is available for consultation and more demanding pupils. Referrals are pointed towards one or the other of these practitioners. The School Home Support workers make home visits, meet parents at school and run sessions for parents. The programme marks the first time that CAMHS workers have had direct access to schools; they work closely with teachers looking at systems for managing children and suggest changes that may improve a particular child's behaviour. By combining home visits and school visits the project has achieved a marked reduction in the levels of emotional behavioural difficulties in pupils.

Extended schools

An 'extended school' essentially means using the school as the base for providing programmes for children and young people beyond learning in the classroom. While many activities may come under the concept, at a minimum it will offer:

- Child care provided through the school site or through school clusters or other local providers. The care provision may last from 8 am to 6pm all year round with supervised transfer arrangements where needed.
- A programme of activities such as homework clubs, study support, sport (two hours beyond the finish of the school day) as well as music, drama and the arts.
- Parenting support including information sessions on childhood transitions and parenting programmes run in collaboration with children's services.
- A swift and easy referral system to a wide range of specialist support such as speech therapy, sexual health, intensive behaviour support and child and adolescent mental health services.

The Education Act 2002 requires schools to consult with pupils, staff, parents and carers, local communities and the local authority to ensure the services they develop are shaped around the needs of the pupils and their local community. Extended schools are not about teachers running services or taking on additional responsibilities. Consistent with the aims of workforce remodelling, schools should ensure only the most appropriate people develop and deliver extended services. For example, support staff may want to be involved as well as external staff such as health and social workers and local sports and arts organisations.

In line with the Children Act 2004, local authorities should be working with key partners to strategically plan, commission and coordinate extended services. This includes helping ensure that all initiatives, such as regeneration, capital programmes for school buildings, the specialist schools initiative, the local children's workforce strategy, local area agreements, children and young people's plans, Sure Start children's centres, link with and support the extended schools agenda.

PROVIDING GENDER BALANCE

Among child care and early education providers the relative absence of men at all levels is striking. The consequence is a relatively homogeneous child care profession which, in the crucial dimension of gender, does not reflect the population it serves. This gender imbalance is compounded by the absence of men in the primary school environment and, somewhat less, in the family environment. In the absence of men in key services for children, boys and girls form their images of men from what they see on their televisions, videos, movies and computer games. Such images rarely depict men as nurturing and frequently show them as violent. To some extent this virtual reality is confirmed by what takes place in the family environment, where domestic violence and oppressive forms of male domination are prevalent.

Children need positive interaction with men in a variety of settings and roles during early childhood. Men may also have a different style of interacting with children, including a more physical style of play, encouraging more independence and a tendency to vary routine over time (Cunningham 1998).

There are enormous practical difficulties in rebalancing gender: the lack of willingness of men to come forward, the heightened sense of risk of sexual abuse that male volunteers might be perceived to bring with them and the possible degree of discomfort for female staff and female volunteers when they have become accustomed to working in a women-centred environment.

Daniel and colleagues note, despite many of the forward-looking developments in early years services, the lack of specific concern with gender issues. They argue for 'gender mainstreaming' in children's services, an approach that recognises that 'policies may impact differently on the lives of women and men, boys and girls, and which attempts to promote gender equity' (Daniel *et al.* 2005: 1344). They cite four issues that should be central to any such mainstreaming:

*   The context of contemporary parenting and many of the suggested lines of action will fall disproportionately on women. *Every Child Matters*, through its use of the word 'parent', pays little attention to the different pressures and positions of mothers and fathers.
*   Women still tend to have primary responsibility for child care but have less access to financial resources.
*   Lone parents are overwhelmingly women and are more vulnerable to poverty and to the conflicting pressure from policy and practice to find work.
*   Women in general bear the brunt of the overt signs of accepting parental responsibility such as home–school contracts and for their children's truanting. Eighty-one per cent of parents attending parenting order programmes were women and half of these were lone parents.

By disregarding gender, early years programmes risk instituting practices unfair to women. These include:

*   identification, referral and tracking schemes will bring increased surveillance (real or perceived) largely focused on mothers; the challenge is to develop systems without increasing pressures on mothers on low incomes
*   The lack of coordination between children's services and adult mental health

services means that, given the association between depression and childcare, women will suffer disproportionately from mental health problems
- reliance on volunteer schemes to provide parent support may founder on lack of sufficient volunteers
- mothers become the sole focus of child maltreatment enquiries.

At the very least, public statements from early years programmes can signal awareness of the importance of male presence in the lives of young children, that the programmes aspire to bring a diversity of approaches to early childhood education and that men will be actively sought to fill caregiver positions within them.

CASE STUDY 5.3: FATHERS' INVOLVEMENT IN SURE START LOCAL PROGRAMMES

Staff in a large majority of Sure Start local programmes reported low levels of father involvement in programme activities. Where fathers took part it was most likely to be in outdoor, active fun-type activities. However, many fathers do have 'arm's length' contact with programmes, through their partners. Fathers are inclined to attend activities designed specifically for them. Events for fathers and children together can be a stepping-stone for fathers into a wider range of Sure Start experiences, including whole family activities.

Most fathers felt welcomed at services provided by Sure Start local programmes, although being in a conspicuous minority among large numbers of women could be daunting, especially at first. Mothers supported the idea of fathers using Sure Start local programme services and of male staff working in them. Fathers continued to come to Sure Start local programme services when they had seen a positive benefit to themselves or their children from a service.

Where programmes had high levels of father involvement, they had decided early in the planning stages of the programme that fathers would be central to their work. In such programmes there was an attempt to spread commitment to fathers to every aspect of the programme and to everyone involved. There was a joined-up approach to involving fathers. An important encouragement for fathers was the presence of a staff member dedicated to involving them. Such workers have helped Sure Start local programmes discover and respond to issues that affect fathers: bereavement and loss, anger management, concerns about child development and feelings of isolation among them.

(Lloyd *et al.* 2003)

KEY POINTS

☐   Neighbourhood environments play a large part in children's development through the resources available and the impact on the choices parents are able to make.

☐   The ecological model is effective in allowing practitioners to capture the different levels of forces that shape a child's life course, including the neighbourhood level.

☐   The framework for the assessment of children in need is based on the ecological model and practitioners are encouraged to give greater prominence to 'the missing side of the triangle' – that part of the framework which deals with neighbourhood conditions.

☐   The comprehensive assessment framework extends beyond issues of need and should be used by all practitioners from any service who work with a particular child so that information is coordinated and intrusion into the child's life is minimal.

☐   The early years are critical to the child's later life course and preventive services should focus first and foremost on children from birth to five.

☐   Schools provide effective hubs for community-based services for children and families.

CHAPTER 6

MEETING THE CHALLENGE OF ANTI-SOCIAL BEHAVIOUR: COMMUNITY-BASED SERVICES FOR YOUNG PEOPLE

OBJECTIVES

By the end of this chapter you should:

- Understand the difficulties in the lengthy period of transition that young people have to negotiate on their way to adulthood

- Become familiar with promising local efforts in services for young people including accelerated crime prevention, school-based inclusion programmes, strengthening networks and improving informal neighbourhood controls

- Be able to think through what anti-social behaviour means in relation to the communities you work in

- Have clarified the role of the 'lead practitioner' in youth support programmes.

This chapter discusses the kinds of services needed to promote the inclusion of young people in their local communities. In particular practice is having to respond to the public's (and government's) concern over anti-social behaviour and 'community safety'. The chapter considers the efforts in localities to rein in anti-social behaviour, reduce crime, and from this platform, develop positive services for young people. This emphasis on anti-social behaviour presents practitioners with a number of dilemmas between using a number of punitive, name-and-shame strategies and the struggle to construct the youth support systems that young people actually require.

TRANSITION TO ADULTHOOD AS CONTEXT FOR PRACTICE

Young people face a range of difficulties now that previous generations did not have to deal with. This new battery of uncertainty and complexity in their lives stems from the lengthy and difficult-to-negotiate transition from youth to adulthood, which sets the context in which practitioners have to work through the many-sided service issues facing them.

In the UK and much of the developed world family arrangements long favoured independent living between the generations. Growing up meant usually leaving the birth family and acquiring the economic independence to form a separate household and family unit. Gaining a foothold in the economy, acquiring the skills or education sufficient for this, and managing relationships with would-be household partner(s) formed a crucial transition point in the life course, one both culturally scripted and structured by economic and social resources (Fussell and Furstenberg 2005).

The entry into adulthood now has become a more drawn out, more complicated process, as a number of observers have shown (Bentley and Gurumurthy 1999; Settersten *et al.* 2005). The very term 'adolescence' was originally coined in the early twentieth century to describe a person on the threshold of adulthood. Now that threshold embraces a wider span of years – starting as early as age twelve and extending to a person's mid-twenties, particularly if still at home and still economically dependent on parents. The traditional markers of adulthood – leaving home, finishing school, starting work, getting married and having children – are, in the words of Furstenberg and colleagues, 'less predictable and more prolonged, diverse and disordered' (Fussell and Furstenberg 2005: 35).

As a result young people in general are often left to face hard and unclear choices. The consequences have been particularly severe on young people from lower-income families. Changes in the economy now prize 'people skills' such as working effectively in teams and knowledge manipulation. This has been accompanied by the drying up of industrial and manufacturing careers which previously provided a steady wage for many years. The consequent emphasis on education, particularly higher education, has increased considerably. Changes in marriage and family patterns have also made the transition to adulthood more difficult: forming first households and sexual partnerships, and the delayed timing within the life course for marriage and having children have brought both greater freedom and confusion. As young adults continue to leave home in their late teens or early twenties they are more likely to establish non-family situations – as single households or in group living. Both trends create ambiguity and uncertainty as to how to achieve the stability, anchorage and the income associated with adulthood. The loss of clear steps and ready markers in the life course of young people should not be underestimated; that loss means turbulent, uncertain years and all who go through it do so with uncertainty and trepidation. For young people from socially excluded housing estates, with parents who do not care, with low incomes or who are homeless, the pressures and uncertainties are ratcheted up further.

Researchers have noted a sharp polarisation in the transition to adulthood. One pathway is taken by substantial numbers of young people who leave school at the minimum age and become parents in their teens. Such transitions are becoming more problematic in the eyes of policymakers and practitioners, and more stigmatised when compared with the middle-class pathway, which defers entry into the labour market and setting up family for many years (Jones 2002). In this process the neighbourhood in which young people live actively shapes the work identities of young men and women. Their work identities are constructed in the first instance *inside* the neighbourhood in response to local gender and ethnic roles. *Outside* perceptions also shape work identities, particularly in lower-income areas where young people are perceived as anti-social, congregating in 'do-nothing' groups, unreliable and uninterested in work (Bauder 2001).

Vulnerable young men, from low-income families and with few qualifications on leaving school, have particular difficulties. Work opportunities for these relatively unskilled workers tended to be temporary and short-term based on sub-contracting or agency employment. They have few chances for training in these casual and insecure sectors and become trapped in precarious patterns which make it difficult for them to secure stable employment (Furlong and Cartmel 2004).

The virtual child: holistic local services across the life span of the young person

One way to achieve interdisciplinary unity around outcomes is to view the range of services that can be provided across the life span of children in a particular neighbour-hood. To do this Paul Boylan, manager of the Neighbourhood Management Pathfinder in Blacon, has devised the model of the 'Virtual Child' that in graphic form highlights the significant risk points a child and young person face. The model shows the kinds of services that are required at different stages in a child's life if, in a given environment, the pressures of that locality – whether poor schooling, adverse peer groups, low income, low-capacity social networks or overcrowded housing – are overwhelming the strengths and resilience of a child and its family.

The Virtual Child was constructed by working backwards from the point when a young male offender reaches his eighteenth birthday in youth custody and then asking how is it that he got there? What services were involved prior to this point and what did they *fail* to do for this outcome to have happened? What would services *not have done* at various risk points of his earlier life in order for him to have ended up in custody? Conversely, what would services have had to do in order to forestall this period in custody? The Virtual Child's life course points to the relative paucity of flexible, alert services in his critical early years, particularly in a family where 'coercive' parenting styles and behaviours were shaping up within the family. It points further to the lack of connection between parents and school, low-capacity peer networks and lack of youth engagement in the labour market (Boylan 2006; Boylan *et al.* 2006).

The Virtual Child

Showing costs of early years and youth services as they respond to challenging and anti-social behaviour in school and community

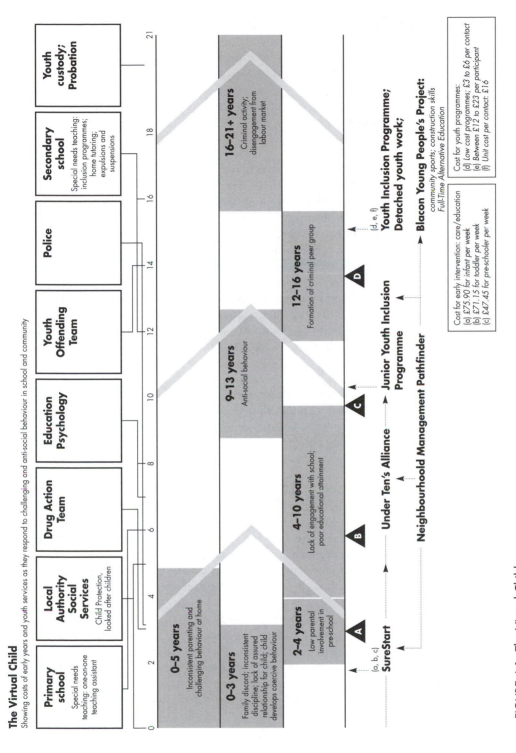

FIGURE 6.1 The Virtual Child

OUTCOMES FOR YOUNG PEOPLE

The green paper from government, *Youth Matters* (DfES 2005b), focuses on what it describes as five key challenges facing services for young people:

- how to engage more young people in positive activities and empower them to shape the services they receive
- how to encourage more young people to volunteer and become involved in their communities
- how to provide better information, advice and guidance to young people to help them make informed choices about their lives
- how to provide better and more personalised intensive support for each young person who has serious problems or gets into trouble
- how to help young people to develop a sense of control and attain some measure of security in their lives to support the transition to adulthood.

The approach of the green paper is governed by a number of underpinning principles which steer agencies towards making services both more responsive to what young people and their parents want and more integrated, efficient and effective by involving a wide range of organisations from the voluntary community and private sectors. In addition to the five outcomes in *Every Child Matters* there are others expressly set out for young people:

- improve a sense of security, self-efficacy and the capacity to plan their future
- secure the assets, or 'human capital', they need to reach adulthood, particularly requisite levels of education
- achieve a sense of well-being and the capacity to form relationships and ultimately households and/or families.

In pursuing these outcomes, services should focus on providing support for the key transitions facing young people such as independent living, finding a place in the world of post-16 education and/or training. This includes helping them to secure a decent income that enables them to make a real choice as to whether to find work or pursue education, and if the former to decide what work they are best suited for.

In helping young people make a successful transition to adulthood, community-based and community-level work with young people forms around four nodes:

- parents and family that offer support and guidance
- working with and through schools to support out of school hours learning or family learning
- strengthening peer networks by drawing on role models, mentoring and volunteers and volunteer activities
- the community's capacity to exert informal controls and limit anti-social behaviour.

**BOX 6.1: WHAT YOUNG PEOPLE NEED TO HELP
WITH THE TRANSITION TO ADULTHOOD**

Research from the Scottish Executive tells us that what disaffected young people need in
programmes are:

•   offered activities which are meaningful and relevant to them and in which they can
    participate on a voluntary basis
•   activities that provide them with a sense of ownership, an alternative learning environment
    from school
•   opportunities for recognising their achievements, and support for transition into other
    education or training
•   practitioner skills to re-engage and motivate disaffected young people; one-to-one support
    is particularly vital in building positive relationships.

(Scottish Executive 2005)

ANTI-SOCIAL BEHAVIOUR AND THE RESPECT AGENDA

Anti-social behaviour has a significant impact on the lives of people living in particular
areas, especially disadvantaged urban neighbourhoods and social housing estates
peripheral to towns and cities. While it dominates government policy and appears as a
widespread problem, in fact only a minority of citizens are affected by it.

Just as there is uncertainty over its actual extent, so there is uncertainty about what
constitutes anti-social behaviour, which the public associates with the actions of young
people such as graffiti writing, congregating in noisy groups on the street and drug
taking. In local neighbourhoods, as Millie and his colleagues discovered, people were
primarily concerned with just three issues: general misbehaviour by children and young
people, visible drug and alcohol misuse and 'problem families' and neighbour disputes
(Millie *et al*. 2005). Public attitudes revealed by that important study indicate a complex
picture at neighbourhood level. Local people tended to see anti-social behaviour as a
sign of social and moral decline and favoured more disciplinary solutions, while local
agencies explained it in terms of social exclusion and deprivation and favoured
prevention and inclusion strategies. In the three case study sites investigated, each had
local strategies in place to combat anti-social behaviour that were graduated and
proportional and balanced preventive services with enforcement (Millie *et al*. 2005).

When talking about the causes of local anti-social behaviour, local people
advanced three different explanations or 'narratives' as to why it happens:

•   social and moral decline: anti-social behaviour seen as a symptom of wider social
    and cultural change, and in particular a decline in moral standards and family
    values
•   disengaged youth and families: anti-social behaviour arises from the increasing

disengagement from the wider society by a significant minority of families and their children

• 'kids will be kids': anti-social behaviour is really the age-old tendency for young people to get into trouble, challenge public and parental boundaries and antagonise their elders (Millie *et al.* 2005).

ACTIVITY 6.1: WHAT IS ANTI-SOCIAL BEHAVIOUR?

Andrew Millie and his colleagues sought out the public's view of what constitutes anti-social behaviour. In their survey they found that a certain percentage of the public thought the following behaviours constituted anti-social behaviour. The list here is presented in no particular order. Rank each behaviour in terms of seriousness and then rate each again in terms of how you think the public at large viewed such behaviours. You can compare your ratings with those of the public by checking the survey results at the back of this volume.

traffic noise and pollution,   rowdy teenagers on the streets/
graffiti,   youths hanging around,
burglary,   noisy neighbours,
vandalism,   mugging,
speeding,   drug dealing.

(Adapted from Millie *et al.* 2005)

Family factors play an important part in possible explanations for youth offending and anti-social behaviour. But it is difficult to disentangle 'family' factors from 'neighbourhood' factors. We know that family variables such as the lack of parental supervision, parental rejection, erratic and harsh discipline, marital conflict, parental crimininality and weak attachment are all significant predictors of anti-social behaviours, including drug use and offending. We know too that protective factors present at different stages of a young person's life provide sources of resilience even in high-risk neighbourhoods: no overcrowding, small families, good maternal health, good home care and parental employment (Haines and Case 2005).

Neighbourhood conditions set the social context in which young people make particular choices. Those that generate temptations in the shape of available commodities and provocations such as insults or threats of violence combine with low levels of social control to present what can be described as 'risk communities' (Wikstrom and Loebner 2000). This context plays out in behaviour settings such as homes, street corners, pubs, outside schools, on school buses or other natural gathering places. As individual young people engage in such settings some will carry highly protective factors such as good parental supervision, high sense of guilt, high motivation in relation to school and a negative perception of anti-social behaviour. Others will carry pronounced risk factors such as attention problems, poor parental supervision, low feelings of guilt, and association with many peer delinquents (Wikstrom and Loebner 2000).

Neighbourhoods' 'efficacy' in maintaining social norms

Risk and protective factors in the neighbourhood are associated with more, or less, informal social controls in neighbourhoods. The notion of neighbourhood 'efficacy' – that is the informal capacity to guide and control the behaviour of residents – has contributed significantly to thinking around what kind of services can reduce levels of anti-social behaviour. Sampson and colleagues found that a sense of mutual trust within a particular neighbourhood provided the subsoil for that efficacy. They found that collective efficacy as a construct can be measured reliably at neighbourhood level and that three dimensions of neighbourhood stratification – concentrated disadvantage, concentrations of new arrivals and residential stability – largely explained why some neighbourhoods were able to exercise sufficient control to inhibit violence and why some were not (Sampson *et al.* 1997). Examples of informal social controls include the monitoring of play groups or teen gatherings, a willingness to intervene to prevent acts such as truancy and littering, and confrontation with persons who are exploiting or disturbing public space (Sampson *et al.* 1997: 918).

BOX 6.2:   THE RESPECT AGENDA

The Respect agenda has adopted the arguments around community processes such as efficacy and the exercise of informal social control, and operationalised them in a particular way. In doing so it has placed greater responsibility on families, communities and neighbourhoods for managing their own disorder and consolidating their informal controls. Community, in the words of Flint, 'becomes both a territory and a means of governing crime and disorder' (Flint 2002: 249).

The rules and patterns of respect mean recognising

that the behaviour of an individual has an effect on the wider society, that we should treat people as we would want to be treated, that we should respect property, privacy and dignity of others, that it is wrong to corrupt the neighbourhood with excessive noise, litter, unruly animals or threatening behaviour, that we should be good neighbours, that children are the responsibility of all adults. These should be self-enforcing.

(Blears 2004: 13)

CASE STUDY 6.1: THE TOGETHER CAMPAIGN

The Home Office's TOGETHER campaign is a reassurance programme in effect responding to what researchers have called the 'signal crimes perspective' – the idea that the reaction of local residents to local 'signal' incidents determines whether or not they fear crime and feel vulnerable. Once identified, so the argument goes, such signal incidents can be countered by 'control signals' that reassure the public (see Innes, 2004 and www.reassurancepolicing.co.uk).

ACTIVITY 6.2:   COLLABORATING IN LOCAL ACTION ON ANTI-SOCIAL BEHAVIOUR

Make a list of the agencies, public and voluntary, together with community organisations and interest groups, in a particular neighbourhood you work in.

Then write beside each of these what you think would be their response to local manifestations of anti-social behaviour. Would you be able to develop a shared definition of what anti-social behaviour is? What would likely be their various explanations of the causes of that behaviour? What actions or interventions do you think they would be willing to adopt or collaborate on in tackling these problems?

This activity is probably best tackled in conjunction with two or three other colleagues and in fact could act as a trigger to forming a 'community of practice' (see Chapter 4) that would form a local strategy.

The situation in communities and neighbourhoods may well be more complex than the Respect agenda (see box) would allow for. The Family and Neighbourhoods Study (FANS) addressed these questions by examining parents' perceptions of their neighbourhood and expectations of their neighbours' behaviour (Barnes 2006a). The neighbourhoods surveyed included a disadvantaged inner city with large minority ethnic population, a socially excluded area of a mid-size town as well as an affluent suburb of a large city. In particular it probed the expectations parents had of informal controls being exercised by their neighbours and whether parents themselves would intervene in particular circumstances. It also sought children's views on this. The study then related these perceptions to the risk and protective factors in each of the very different neighbourhoods surveyed.

The findings showed that several powerful variables are at work clustered around the degree of affluence of a neighbourhood. In the more affluent neighbourhoods there was greater confidence about shared parenting norms even if neighbours did not know each other very well. On the other hand when neighbours were known and parenting values were known, shared informal control was more likely to exist. In the one affluent area surveyed this presumption was widely held by residents (Barnes 2006a).

In the highly disadvantaged neighbourhood, on the other hand, parents expected to be ignored or verbally abused when they attempted to exercise control. Fear of retaliation/retribution for any intervention related to low levels of local agreement about parenting and low levels of attachment to the neighbourhood in which they were resident, and was more likely to be felt by those less attached to their neighbourhood and those who rate the neighbourhood of poor quality. Aggressive parenting styles were now more openly displayed within schools, sports events and youth centres. In general parents tended to think that neighbours would intervene for the common good and set standards for behaviour in the neighbourhood. However, this was tempered by uncertainty as to whether parents are like-minded, and suspicions that they may not be (Barnes 2006a).

BOX 6.3: PARENTS' AND OLDER CHILDREN'S VIEWS OF INFORMAL SOCIAL CONTROLS IN AFFLUENT AND DISADVANTAGED NEIGHBOURHOODS

'I just think the people, generally speaking, are decent people. *We are all like minded* and I think we all look out for one another's children as well.' (Italics in original.)

'It was within a cul-de-sac and from what I gathered *all my neighbours there were of the same thinking*. We all looked out for other people's children.' (Italics in original.)

'The kids aren't very nice, put it that way, a lot of the kids aren't very nice in this area any more. I won't walk past them on my own at night time, put it that way.'

'Their teenage kids hang outside here all night. You tell them to keep the noise down and you get abuse back. You hear them screaming round in cars. You report it to the police and they don't want to know. It gets me down and it's a big worry with the children.'

(All quotes taken from Barnes 2006a)

ACTIVITY 6.3: HOW LIKELY WOULD NEIGHBOURS BE TO INTERVENE IF . . .?

In assessing how much informal control a particular neighbourhood has over the behaviour of young people, much depends on the *perception* of those who live there and the willingness of parents themselves to intervene.

The FANS study (see above) asked specific questions of individuals about whether they would intervene when faced with particular behaviours by children in their neighbourhood. Researchers asked local people whether their neighbours would be likely to intervene with a five- or six-year-old child who was misbehaving, or with a young person engaging in delinquent acts, or to assist a child deemed at risk.

Drawing on the list from that study, what would your personal response be to these behaviours by a five- or six-year-old?

Has a knife;
taking something from house, garage or garden;
playing with matches;
spray paints or writes on a building or car;
left alone in the evening; throws rocks at another child;
left alone during the day; shoplifting;
falls off a bike; throws rocks at a dog; wandering by him/herself;
hits a child the same age; being spanked by an adult in the street;
picks flowers from a garden.

Rate your response for each on a scale of 1 to 5 with 1 indicating that intervention by adults is very unlikely to 5 where intervention is very likely. Then do the same for what you think the response would be in general from adults in your neighbourhood. When complete consult the survey answers at the back of this volume.

Practitioners working in parents' or neighbourhood groups could use these questions to engage in a discussion on these matters:

- What are parents' responsibilities, what are neighbourhood norms, and what are the grounds for intervening in events involving other people's children?
- How to solidify positive peer and friendship groups.
- Identify safe places to meet.
- How might local social participation and 'active citizenship' programmes improve knowledge about neighbours?
- Greater facilities for young people to meet in the locality where informal controls prevail.

EMOTIONAL HEALTH AND RESILIENCE

There is increasing practitioner interest in the concept of 'resilience' and in 'emotional intelligence' or emotional health. Many children survive difficult family life, poor parenting and, even abuse to emerge as adults leading fulfilling lives. Equally, although there is a pronounced link between disadvantage in childhood and subsequent poverty in adulthood, there is a noted capacity to emerge from disadvantage without health, behavioural, learning or emotional problems. That many children do survive challenging environments raises the question why some do and others do not. Practitioners have had the tendency to see the young person emerging from disadvantage or the child coping with adverse parenting as 'vulnerable' and as having 'needs' so that their perspectives are guided by children most at risk. There is the danger here of a community perspective based on concepts of vulnerability, risk and high levels of need rather than focusing on the elements that promote emotional health.

Much rests on the individual child's own capacity to escape from disadvantage. Psychologists' evidence points to certain characteristics: a strong relationship with a dependable caregiver, reasonable level of self-confidence, sense of control and optimism, and the capacity to reflect and to solve problems and to hold aspirations for the future. Children cope with adversity if they have developed certain social or emotional skills – in this the influential role played by a strong relationship between a child and a significant caring adult is critical, with work to support that parenting role when necessary (Harker 2005).

Building a young person's resilience and capacity to overcome adversity places the emphasis on developing a network of support from the resources available across all three levels of the child's social ecology, including the neighbourhood and community, and relatively less emphasis on professional intervention. Daniel and Wassell (2002) have based their entire approach to assessment and intervention on six domains of resilience that cut across the three levels of the ecological model: individual, family and community. These are:

- the young person's social competencies
- a secure base for the young person
- educational achievements
- friendships
- talents and interest
- positive values.

Factors within each of these, and at each of the three levels of the ecological model, contribute to a child's level of either vulnerability or resilience (Daniel and Wassell 2002). Their valuable handbook for working with adolescents presents a number of ready questions that will help the practitioner probe each of these dimensions.

BOX 6.4: DANIEL AND WASSELL'S CHECKLIST FOR ASSESSING A YOUNG PERSON'S RESILIENCE IN EDUCATION

The first group of questions probes the young person's views on school, the second group her or his family's attitudes to school, and third group the views of the young person on what support they might find in the wider community.

Young person's views on school

- Why do you think young people have to go to school?
- What do you think of your school? If you could change anything in your school what would it be?
- Do you find you can concentrate in class? If not why do you think that is?
- What is your favourite subject? Your least favourite subject?
- Who would you go to if you did not understand something in your favourite subject? In your least favourite subject?

continued

Young person's views on family support for education

- Who do you think takes an interest in your school progress?
- How much do your parents and/or carers know about your progress in school?
- Do you have a private place to study?
- Who helps you with homework?
- Who goes to parents' evenings and who would you like to go?

Young person's views on sources of support in community

- Do you meet up with any of the other young people at school?
- Is there anyone else that you know outside school who can help you with your studying?
- Do you go to any learning or homework clubs?
- Is there any teacher that you feel you have a good relationship with?

(Daniel and Wassell 2002: 40–41)

IMPULSIVITY AND BEHAVIOUR PROBLEMS

There is a rising tide of behavioural difficulties in schools, pre-schools and neighbourhoods, with much popular and professional speculation as to cause and effect – from the triple jab, video games, television and food additives to parental laxness and non-existent community controls. Conduct disorders and impulsivity – two concepts researched at length by psychologists and child psychiatrists – capture some of the disruptive effects of an entire spectrum of behaviours. Impulsive behaviour – apparently spontaneous, unpremeditated and wilful – stems from the young person's or child's restlessness, impatience and inability to concentrate. Conduct disorders, as defined by child psychologists, are those behaviours in children deemed provocative and coercive. They typically include bullying, tantrums, truancy, shoplifting, physical assault, lying, cruelty to animals, vandalism or destruction of home or school property. Clearly there are strong parallels between conduct disorders and anti-social behaviour.

Conduct problems develop from an accumulation of multiple experiences rather than from a single environmental determinant (Rutter *et al.* 1998). Any model for understanding the complexity of effects must be able to accommodate the effects of neighbourhood disadvantage and the stresses affecting parenting styles, the role of siblings and peers, and the individual personality traits of the child.

There is also a large increase in young people with mental health problems compared with numbers in the 1970s. The proportion of young people with conduct problems more than doubled to 15 per cent in 1999, and increases in emotional problems between 1986 and 1999 rose from 10 to 17 per cent (Collinshaw *et al.* 2004). Rates of self-harm among young people in Britain are among the highest in Europe. Yet services promoting emotional well-being in children are developing slowly. The role schools play in educating young people about mental health has thus far been highly restricted. Children and adolescent mental health services are oversubscribed with long waiting lists and uneven provision. Services for young people with acute or severe mental illness are often lacking, with few beds and delays or inappropriate admission to adult beds.

Lower levels of informal controls as discussed above present a context in which impulsive behaviour by young people, mainly male, is allowed to become more prominent in its impact. This can happen in one of two ways: either it may increase the opportunities for crime – 'where opportunity is defined as the coming together in time and space of a potential perpetrator with a potential victim in the absence of public guardians', or the informal controls are 'external' and are missed by those young people who have few 'internal' – or self–controls (Lynam *et al.* 2000: 571). However, for young people with sufficient self control in place, residence in disadvantaged neighbourhoods in and of itself did not appear to stimulate higher levels of offending.

Many programmes are aimed at helping parents enhance the 'prosocial' behaviours of their offspring such as Webster-Stratton's Incredible Years (Webster-Stratton 1992) and the Positive Parenting Programme (Triple P). Careful evaluation has demonstrated their effectiveness (Martin and Sanders 2003). Such programmes centre largely on the transactions between parents and offspring; few take into account the neighbourhood contexts in which the families reside. To do this, Brody and colleagues suggest that to improve the effectiveness of such programmes it is necessary to involve grandparents and other extended-family caregivers of a child with behavioural difficulties and to provide them with the means of monitoring that child's behaviour at school. Such programmes decrease what Patterson and colleagues (2000) call 'wandering' – the unsupervised time in which the opportunistic contact with anti-social peers takes place – thereby lessening the likelihood of engaging in anti-social behaviour (cited in Brody *et al.* 2003).

There is a difference between high levels of monitoring and control and a parenting style that is both harsh and inconsistent and that has long been associated with conduct disorder in boys. In the latter, frequent episodes of hitting, shouting and abrupt withdrawal are associated with ever-escalating 'coercive behaviours' and can be further intensified by older sibling behaviour (Patterson 1992). Brody and colleagues have uncovered an extremely important finding that underscores the power of neighbourhood effect: younger siblings engaged in anti-social behaviour when an older sibling had greater deviance-prone tendencies *and* the family resided in a disadvantaged neighbourhood. There was no such link in families who did not reside in disadvantaged neighbourhoods (Brody *et al.* 2003: 219).

WORKING WITH SCHOOLS ON YOUTH INCLUSION

As extended schools become a service hub (see Chapter five) there is considerable scope for non-teaching, school-based support workers of various kinds. Increasingly they work together with schools to reduce school exclusions and provide family support and other programme aims. It has become clearer that teaching staff have neither the time nor the training to carry this work out effectively. While school-attached social workers may be regarded by education colleagues as external and not really focused on school ethos, the demands of the curriculum, pressure from league tables, problems of pupil selection and enrolment have simply meant that teachers are unable to perform the pastoral roles originally outlined in efforts to minimise school exclusions.

Inclusion coordinators offer a good example of the direction that such work is heading. It calls on skills both familiar and new to social workers: crisis intervention, listening, using assessment frameworks in an educational setting and using social services databases among others. Developing new elements to the role assists improvement in how teachers and school management regard family link-work. Inclusion coordinators assist education partners and other agencies in developing responses to behaviour with which they are unfamiliar, such as Asperger's syndrome, domestic violence or mental health problems. Located within children's services, inclusion coordinators can form the cornerstone of family and school support teams, which may include social workers, family support workers, police, youth workers, educational psychologists, mental health workers, school nurses and education welfare or education inclusion officers.

CASE STUDY 6.2: THE MATRIX PROJECT

The Matrix Project in Dorset aimed to reduce anti-social behaviour by children ages 8 to 11 by working with the whole family and drawing in other services including mental health, debt and advice. Sponsored by the Dorset Health Alliance Project, it reduced school exclusions in an area where they were rife by providing a social work service for children and families in primary schools linked to a secondary school. Astounding results: the project halved the truancy rate, brought about a reduction in delinquency and improved teachers' morale and high levels of educational attainment by pupils.

(adapted from Pugh and Statham 2006)

Another example of evolving roles outside of the teaching staff but within schools is found in 'into work' programmes which are often aimed at young men who are disengaged from the national curriculum and indeed on the edges of school altogether. This requires greater flexibility on the part of schools in their approach to life-related, non-academic programmes. The programmes respond by arranging workplace visits and treating participants as responsible adults and expecting them to behave accordingly.

Such programmes emphasise interview experience, using the telephone, completion of CVs and application forms, exploration of training options on leaving school, where and how to look for jobs, what it is like being part of a workforce and discussion of career and job options. The approach encourages individual exploration rather than information retention and builds young men's confidence, helping them to think and find out for themselves. This in turn calls for specific skills in engaging young men in life-focused learning and relationship building (Lloyd *et al.* 2002).

YOUTH OFFENDING AND DRUG MISUSE

Drug misuse by young people has damaging ecological effects. The associated patterns of behaviour are multiple: damage to the health of individuals, damage to peer networks, theft from neighbours or family members, loss of aspiration and pain for the victims of drug-related crime as well as other family members of the offender.

Restorative justice techniques are a promising, neighbourhood-based response to the teenage heroin abuser who commits a burglary.* In the restorative justice process all those who have been affected by the crime come together to discuss how to restore both materially and psychologically the damage done. It is a supremely local response to offending that occurs in the midst of the neighbourhood. Its aim is to secure recognition from the young offender of the injustice arising from his or her dependency: understanding that stealing from friends and family and lying and other untrustworthy behaviour cause immense hurt. Often the victims of the crime are family members and 'bear the burden of injustice out of love for the offender' (Braithwaite 2001: 228). This, argues Braithwaite, is contingent on empathy and love for the offender that in turn is the source of motivation for the offender in his or her wish to discard the dependency and to see healed both the substance abuse and the injustice that it caused (Braithwaite 2001: 229). Restorative justice circles also allow the offender to contest or refute a charge made. From this deliberative element involving discussion on all sides of the offence the process builds a democratic commitment to carrying out the agreed acts of restoration. Braithwaite sees wide application of the approach to, for example, drunk and dangerous driving and family violence, which may also be related to forms of dependency. This response of a local circle to a crime often provides the launch point for change – the call for help from parents, the wish of the offender to discard his old self. It may also be the chance to turn a private trouble into a public issue by campaigning for drug law reform, greater rehabilitative options or stricter speed limits at dangerous road crossing points (Braithwaite 2001).

CASE STUDY 6.3: BLACON COMMUNITY SAFETY PARTNERSHIP AND YOUTH PARTNERSHIP WORK IN RELATION TO DRUG MISUSE

Blacon is a large social housing estate on the edge of Chester with some 15,000 residents. With the Neighbourhood Management Pathfinder on the estate acting as broker and catalyst, it has pioneered a number of successful community initiatives. In responding to the dilemmas presented by anti-social behaviour – on the one hand vigorous local opinion wanting something to be done, on the other the realisation that preventive and inclusive action is the most effective way to tackle it – a wide ranging youth inclusion programme has been established.

Work began with a community safety survey that revealed that 69 per cent of residents in Blacon over the age of 16 thought that drugs were easy to get in the area (compared with a response rate of 44 per cent among residents in Chester district). In the same survey, 30 per cent of 14- and 15-year-olds reported frequently seeing drug 'paraphernalia' around. This data suggests that the use of illegal drugs in the Blacon area was widespread and growing.

continued

---

* I am indebted to a highly persuasive article on this subject by John Braithwaite of the Australian National University. See Braithwaite 2001.

A subsequent audit revealed that current monitoring processes were not providing sufficiently accurate or detailed information needed to deliver targeted services: data concerning the number of detected offences in Blacon relating to drug supply and drug possession recorded only two offences in 2005. These figures were impossibly low and did not reflect the actual supply or use of drugs in the Blacon area. By drawing on local knowledge the data became more precise. For example, syringe exchange services in a Blacon pharmacy had a total of 66 clients, and in addition it is known that other users attend a drug rehab service in Chester, where some192 Blacon residents were registered.

The conclusion was reached that the police had other priorities such as burglary, vehicle crime and violent crime. Tackling drug supply was moreover not included as a key performance indicator for the police within the Police Performance and Assessment Framework. In addition, that part of the government's Drug Intervention Programme concerned with getting drug users out of crime and into treatment appears not to be achieving a high level of success in the Chester area, partly because there is no current practice of drug testing of arrestees for all crime.

Work focusing especially on youth has included DISC (Drugs Intervention Service – Cheshire) that provides substance misuse advice and information to young people and youth organisations as well as undertaking intensive one-to-one work with individuals. A variety of other projects concerned with drug information and education have been provided through day events and short courses delivered by Blacon U Project, Delta Centre, Blacon Young People's Project and Blacon Junior Youth Inclusion Project. Approximately 150 older children and teenagers have been involved in these various projects, as well as a variety of health agencies including community drugs teams, Turning Point Residential Detox and Residential Rehabilitation. All initiatives and services are being delivered in accordance with the government's *National Drugs Strategy: Tackling Drugs to Build a Better Britain* (DfES 2002) as well as within the clear intentions of the green paper *Youth Matters* (DfES 2005b).

There are several important lessons in this case study. First, the right data is crucial; while official information will be available and often useful it *must* be supplemented by local knowledge, that is local databases and information held by residents and local community services. Second, convening local stakeholders – those interested in developing a solution to the problem – is essential. Once together, the task is to arrive at joint definitions of the problem and to harmonise perspectives on the problem, canvassing possible solutions and allocating responsibilities and actions. Third, successful neighbourhood partnerships such as this require strong intermediaries. Bringing together a wide variety of organisations is not easy; it requires brokerage skills and the capacity for patient negotiation, fortunately in this instance provided by Neighbourhood Management Pathfinder personnel.

CASE STUDY 6.4: PRISON VISIT FOR YOUNG PEOPLE

A young person's centre, in collaboration with the Cheshire Youth Federation, developed a short programme to educate young people at risk of anti-social behaviour about prison life. Its aim was to de-romanticise being made subject of an ASBO and to get the young boys involved to look hard at what going to prison actually means.

The session was in two parts. The first, held in the young person's centre, asked the group to fill out a basic worksheet about what their feelings about crime and their knowledge of prison. (Some of the responses by the boys to those questions are included in brackets; in general these revealed startling ignorance about prison life and were laced with profanities and aggression.) The second part of the programme was based on a visit to prison.

The questions concerning prison

What would you miss most in the outside world? ('Booze, chocolate, being free, cars, family, friends, girlfriend')

Who would come to visit you? ('Family, people, friends')

Who would you miss the most? ('Mum, dad, sister, dog, girlfriend')

Who would miss you the most? ('Family, mum, dad')

What would you earn in prison? ('£150 per week, £2 per week')

Can you have money sent in by friends/family? ('Yes')

Will you have a television in your room? ('Yes')

Can you get married in prison, have a baby or attend a funeral? ('Yes')

Other questions probed the young men's feeling about crime and punishment

What would you do and how would you feel if . . .

Someone stole one of your possessions, such as a mobile phone? ('Batter him and rob him'; 'I would punch him and never speak to him'; 'Kick em in an rob his phone'.)

Someone threw rubbish into your front garden? ('Say something to him and tell him you do it again and I'll make you eat it'; 'Chuck it in there garden'; 'I would make them eat it and be pissed off'.)

Someone wrecked your prize possession? ('Wreck something of theirs'; 'Really annoyed'; 'Break his face'.)

Someone constantly kept you awake all night with loud music or arguing? ('Go around their house'; 'Really annoyed'.)

Someone constantly pushed into you when passing you and was constantly calling you names? ('Asked them what there problem was – not that bothered'; 'Hit them'; 'Have a fight – I be pissed off'.)

Someone drove so badly that you were injured because of it? ('Run them over – it's only fair if they have done it to me'; 'Rob the car'; 'Tell them [the Courts] to take there license again'.)

CASE STUDY 6.5: HEALTH EDUCATION FOR LIFE PROJECT

HELP is an action research project in Liverpool. It reveals the not surprising finding that adolescents prefer to turn to their friends rather than talk to professionals. But more than that the

continued

project has developed strategies for helping young people to cope with transitions and frustrations. It provides specialist staff such as learning mentors and counsellors who take on pastoral roles that teachers do not have time for. It also assists young people in finding other ways to express themselves through the arts.

Regular audits of young people in the criminal justice system show that reasons for offending behaviour are lifestyle and peer emulation, abuse, poor parenting and social exclusion – very similar to reasons for mental health and drug problems. Nacro has reported that one-third of 16 to 18-year-olds sentenced by courts have a primary mental disorder including learning disabilites. Half of males on remand and about one-third of young men sentenced have a diagnosable disorder. Frequent drug use is a problem in all these groups and their health needs are not being met (Nacro 1999).

CASE STUDY 6.6: WALTHAM FOREST YOUTH OFFENDING TEAM

Young people often find it difficult to approach mental health services. With young offenders or those at risk of offending this is compounded by the lack of sensitivity and outreach by practitioners in the criminal justice system. Waltham Forest Youth Offending Team (YOT) has sought to overcome this by training members of the team in basic screening techniques for discerning mental health problems. The team offers this to other local agencies working with young people as well: magistrates, school nurses and the fire brigade (to enable it to deal more expertly with young arsonists). The objective is to ensure that young people with mental health problems who are at risk of offending are diverted from the criminal justice system and seen by specialists within mental health services quickly.

Monthly interagency meetings between Waltham YOT and the Children and Adolescent Mental Health Service take place to discuss specific young people who could not be sectioned under the Mental Health Act but who have severe mental health and drug problems. In such cases the YOT court reports call for community-based sentences rather than custodial ones, with more specialised psychiatric reports available if custody is imminent.

The team found that general health assessments showed that many young people with mental health difficulties had not seen a GP and that simply by registering them with a GP opened up the way to further health services. The YOT's premises were used by GPs holding clinics, school nurses delivering vaccinations and giving advice on contraception, diet, hygiene and health. Addressing health problems allowed for further progress on mental health. It also enabled opportunities to build therapeutic relationships at the point of highest need, such as arrest, receiving custodial sentence, parents' separation or mental illness.

(Adapted from Smith 2005)

LEAVING INSTITUTIONS AND RESETTLING IN THE COMMUNITY

The child welfare, special education and youth justice systems have a profound effect on the transition to adulthood – adding, in the words of Settersten, 'burdens of stigma and alienation to young adults who already bring low personal and social capital to this juncture' (Settersten 2005: 545). For a large percentage of young people leaving public systems such as young offenders institutions, care or special education, the task of resettling in the community is compounded by limited life skills, health problems, and emotional and behavioural problems. In the US 30 per cent of young people leaving the care system are unprepared to manage their own budget, live on their own, know how to obtain housing or find a job. Moreover, learning disability is prominent among young people in all three systems. For example, in the youth correctional system in the US it is estimated that between 30 per cent and 50 per cent of all youth have an identified learning disability (Foster and Gifford 2005).

Difficult transitions for young people looked after by the local authority

Often the sheer gravity of the situation in which young people leaving care find themselves is muted for practitioners unaware of the wider picture of barriers and deficits care leavers face, with lack of educational attainment among the most prominent.

In 2005 there were some 61,000 children looked after by local authorities in the UK. Of these 27 per cent had a statement of educational need, compared to three per cent of the overall population. Among care leavers only 44 per cent of looked-after children at age 11 achieved the expected level of educational attainment compared with 80 per cent nationally. At 16 only one in ten achieved five or more GCSEs at grades A–C, compared to more than half of all children. Across the board they do not receive adequate help with emotional, mental and physical health and well-being (Social Exclusion Unit 2003). The reasons for what might be termed this 'careless deschooling' have been known for some time: changes in placement interrupt schooling so that looked-after children miss a substantial number of days in school because they do not have a place in a school, have been excluded from school, attend non-mainstream settings or are educated in the home. Often a lack of support from schools themselves combines with a lack of support for learning and development by carers in their placement (Jackson 1998). Some 2,900 unaccompanied asylum-seeking children who were looked after in 2005 faced additional and particular burdens of their own in achieving independence.

But lack of educational attainment is not the only deficit. In 2003 45 per cent of looked after children had a conduct, hyperactivity or emotional disorder compared to 10 per cent of the child population as a whole. (HM Treasury, DfES and DWP 2003; HM Treasury and DfES 2005). In the US between 30 and 40 per cent of children in foster care had physical or emotional problems or some identifiable psychosocial disorder. In one American residential facility researchers also found a strikingly high level of poor health: more acute injuries (broken bones, head injuries, wounds), more physical discomfort, more chronic disorders, lower self-esteem (Foster and Gifford 2005).*

Suitable accommodation remains a chief priority for care leavers and as a means for achieving a successful transition to adulthood. Despite the Children (Leaving Care) Act 2000, which put in place 'pathway plans' for care leavers to be overseen by local authorities, many young care leavers have had to spend lengthy time in bed and breakfast accommodation before designated flats became available. There was evidence too that such holding accommodation was often found in unsafe neighbourhoods (Morgan 2006). In such areas skills for living are more, not less, important yet the average age of young people when they leave care for independence is 16 or 17 (unchanged from twenty or even thirty years ago) while for the population as a whole the age is 23.

Beyond a necessary focus on housing, mentoring systems have also proved their worth in assisting care leavers in their transition to independence. Mentoring relationships, whether one-to-one with a volunteer adult or through peer mentoring groups, allowed care leavers to draw on a new line of support, separate from professional systems or family. Mentoring is both instrumental – allowing the negotiation and realisation of personal goals – and expressive – allowing for befriending and emotional support (Clayden and Stein 2005).

ACTIVITY 6.4: EDUCATIONAL ATTAINMENT OF LOOKED-AFTER YOUNG PEOPLE

Public Service targets set by the Social Exclusion Unit in 2003 aimed at cutting the gap by 2006:

- outcomes in English and maths for looked-after 11-year-olds must be 60 per cent as good as the results of their peers
- no more than 10 per cent of looked-after young people reach school leaving age without having sat a GCSE exam or equivalent
- the proportion of those aged 16 who gain five GCSEs or equivalent at grades A–C must have risen on average by four percentage points each year since 2002.

Dig out the necessary information for your locality and discover whether or not the Public Service targets have been met.

---

* An excellent research network focusing on the vulnerabilities of young people in the care system is the Research Network on Transitions to Adulthood and Public Policy, funded by the MacArthur Foundation and based at the University of Pennsylvania in Philadelphia http://www.transad.pop.upenn.edu/.

Resettling young offenders

A Youth Justice Board report found that 40 per cent of the young offenders (18 years or younger) they surveyed had been homeless or were badly housed while some 75 per cent had lived with persons other than their parents. These figures compare against a national average for this age group, who have lived with persons other than their parents or who have been homeless, of 1.5 per cent. For those in custody some 26 per cent did not know where they would be spending their first night on release (Youth Justice Board 2007). We know that good housing plays an important role in young offenders' lives: a Social Exclusion Unit report found that good housing can reduce re-offending by up to 20 per cent (SEU 2002). Placing young offenders in poor accommodation on release damages their transition to independence.

ACTIVITY 6.5: HOMELESSNESS AND YOUNG OFFENDERS

In 2004 15 per cent of young offenders coming out of custody were left homeless after their local authorities failed to house them. As a result of figures of that sort the Youth Justice Board is looking to phase out placing young offenders in bed and breakfast by 2010 (Youth Justice Board 2006). If you work with young people, how do you think your agency could participate in such a strategy? What specific steps could you take as a practitioner? Do you see the housing of young offenders on release from youth custody as a community issue or a service issue?

STREET-BASED YOUTH WORK IN DEPRIVED COMMUNITIES

Where street-based or detached youth work projects exist they have been found to be remarkably effective. A recent extensive survey of projects reaching some 65,000 young people showed that detached youth work had moved towards short-term work with higher-risk groups, particularly socially excluded youth, over 30 per cent of whom were not in education or employment and over 45 per cent of whom had a history of offending (Crimmens *et al.* 2004). As the researchers discovered, one of the key dynamics to young people gathering on the streets is that the relatively few who have high needs are associating with those with low needs or low risk. The strategy of the workers is often to work with this latter group, who then provide potentially powerful influence and support systems to those young people with high needs.

In a little-known story, these street-based projects delivered impressive results. Those young people in the projects not in work or education or training fell from 29 per cent to 21 per cent three to four months later; those considered to be a core member of groups engaged in anti-social activity fell from 18 per cent to 4 per cent; regular attendance in structured activity rose from 26 per cent to 37 per cent; the numbers sleeping rough fell from 7 per cent to 1.5 per cent (Crimmens *et al.* 2004).

The projects served as an important source of information on work or training for groups of young people who had lost contact with all other agencies. But even more important is the relational aspect, the role modelling, the mentoring and the discussion about norms and boundaries that takes place within any youth work. Detached youth work is conducted away from youth centres or schools and generally on the home territory of young people. What is striking is the capacity of the workers to build relationships and a sense of mutual trust. This takes time and can work in surprising ways in slowly introducing into the young person's life what social relationships mean and how conduct is based on regard for the needs of others.

The same study, however, reported that for many workers a tension existed between the shorter-term, target-based impact which government and funders were expecting and the time needed to develop relationships and the long-term support that was still required from workers (Crimmens *et al.* 2004).

COMMUNITY NAVIGATOR: THE 'LEAD PROFESSIONAL'

Increasingly young people's services are turning to the concept of a 'lead professional' to coordinate and interlink the multiple services for young people. A cross between a case manager and key worker, the lead professional assumes major responsibilities not only for integrating the services for a particular young person but for being the key point of contact.

CASE STUDY 6.7: LEAD PROFESSIONAL FOR THE CUNNINGHAMS

Marcia, the mother, is 38, on her own, and grew up in care. She has three children: Stacy 11, Justin, 14, and Joe, 19. All three truant regularly from school and each has been excluded from school on more than one occasion for disruptive behaviour in the classroom. Joe left school without any qualifications and has appeared before youth justice panels for stealing and vandalism. Stacy has seen various doctors for what is seen by the school nurses as possible depression while Justin has been diagnosed as having attention deficit and hyperactivity disorder.

The list of professionals involved with this family is as follows:

- two school nurses
- two different social workers (from different teams: adolescent support team, and child assessment)
- three educational welfare officers
- two personal advisers from the Connexions youth service
- two workers from the youth offending team
- two educational psychologists

- one substance misuse worker
- three GPs from the family's local surgery
- two child mental health workers (CAMHS)
- one housing officer

Total: 20 professionals.

What is striking is how the different needs of the family revealed themselves over time and have escalated in severity, yet none of the services were able to ameliorate the family's difficulties. As each service became involved a different assessment was conducted : each child referred from service to service and assessed by each. Work duplicated, and time wasted.

A lead professional liked and trusted by the family was chosen to oversee the work of all the services. The role had three responsibilities: to act as a single point of contact for the family; to work as a broker for the different services as they sought to meet the needs of the individual children; to ensure the right help was delivered.

In greater Manchester the local authority in Trafford now gives some lead professionals their own budget to commission services directly. The role has been particularly effective within schools, with parents now being listened to by one person.

A lead professional may be a social worker, mental health worker or member of youth offending team, or a teacher, learning mentor or health visitor. Clearly schools will be principal site for their base. Contradictions in the role may emerge, particularly whether budget holding is consistent with the coordinator role. The lead professional may act as a trusted navigator to help a family find their way through the system. But families may also expect this to include a level of advocacy with the gatekeepers to resources. The lead professional cannot carry out this part of the role if they are themselves one of those gatekeepers – and in some cases the main, or only, gatekeeper (BASW 2006).

KEY POINTS

- [ ] Young people face a complex, difficult transition into adulthood. This is particularly so for socially excluded young people, young people in need and those who have been looked after by the local authority or in the juvenile justice system and young people who have had mental health problems.

- [ ] Government policy on anti-social behaviour has emphasised neighbourhoods and communities taking responsibility for exerting informal social controls. It has also emphasised deterrent measures in relation to anti-social behaviour by young people. These policies present both dilemmas and opportunities for social workers engaged in community practice.

- [ ] A range of new pathways for practice are opening up: school inclusion programmes and street-based youth work among others.

- [ ] The concept of the 'lead professional' is a highly demanding role combining high levels of ability to relate well with young people with negotiating, coordinating and navigating skills with a range of youth services.

CHAPTER 7

COMMUNITIES THAT CARE: DIGNITY AND WELL-BEING FOR OLDER PEOPLE

OBJECTIVES

By the end of this chapter you should:

- Know the outcomes for older people that services should aim for

- Be able to promote neighbourhood-based resources in order to achieve those outcomes

- Become familiar with the recent initiatives in services for older people: the national service framework, intermediate care, and single assessment process

- Understand the importance of networks in delivering care and the links between network based care and the local community.

The phrase 'older people' is common place in social work, social care and health care for the good reason that it is less stigmatising than the alternatives. It is difficult to say precisely at what age a person becomes 'older' but that is the point: it is a relative designation that allows for flexibility of application and a great range of capacities and competences. As a result it is more inclusive and does not stigmatise the way the phrases 'old people' or 'the elderly' do. While one could say that in general the term applies to people of state pensionable age (for men at 65, women at 60) it usually refers to people older than that. As a rough rule of thumb, from the age of 70 onwards individuals may well be regarded as 'older' in certain dimensions of their life – as a parent or driver for example – without being considered so in other areas, such as consumer of health care, jazz musician, religious leader or judge. The different aspects of identity and functioning only differentially become 'older' as the person's life course progresses.

OLDER PEOPLE AND SOCIAL EXCLUSION

The degree of social exclusion experienced by older people is closely linked to the places they live. We know that transitions and major life events play a major role in paring away familial relationships and neighbourhood friendships for older people. Losing a partner, adjusting to living alone, loss of close family members and friends, withdrawal from the labour market, onset of chronic illness and disability come together in powerful sequence. Such events heighten the sense of exclusion and often produce a changed perception of physical safety and harm from crime.

The Social Exclusion Unit's report on the exclusion of older people in disadvantaged neighbourhoods (SEU 2005) underscored the significance of 'neighbourhood' in the exclusionary process. It uncovered in particular the extent to which older people 'age in place', that is spend the greater part of their lives in the same community, and were able to chart the changes to their immediate locality. The report also identified that older people were vulnerable to changes in the character of the neighbourhood through resident turnover, economic decline, or the rise in anti-social behaviour and feelings of insecurity.

The SEU report mapped five elements through which older people experience multiple exclusion from:

- basic services
- material resources
- civic participation
- social relations
- the neighbourhood itself.

Of these the exclusion most commonly experienced by older people fell into the category of 'social relations', which included such factors as isolation and loneliness, and lack of participation in everyday social activities. Exclusion from material resources was the second most widely experienced. The SEU report went further to note how the forms of exclusion combine to form powerful barriers to well-being in the lives of older people (Scharf *et al.* 2005).

Exclusion of older people relates to the ecological definition of neighbourhood proposed in this volume – social relations, civic participation and neighbourhood itself are all tied to 'place' and what happens to people in that place. For example, loss of nearby friends or family for a person who has lived a long time in a single place is often the catalyst for that person viewing their locality in a different light. Older people who held very negative views of their neighbourhood, who felt unsafe for example going out after dark, was another indication of exclusion from the neighbourhood.

Thus the neighbourhood plays a major role in older people's sense of self and identity and in shaping the quality of their daily lives (Scharf 2002). Views on change, degree of resident turnover, the alteration to physical environment and parallel decline in trust of neighbours may merge together to form a generalised sense of insecurity and threat, even when the older person has not been a victim of crime.

BOX 7.1: OLDER PEOPLE VOICE THEIR FEELINGS ABOUT EXCLUSION

'If anyone comes in to me and sit down and talk I'm glad. But then if they don't invite me in their house, I don't want to go. . . . Maybe they would like to have me, but they don't invite me.'

'When you are elderly no one comes to see if you are all right. I mean there should be a welfare officer that knocks at the door. . . . We don't get help here. No one comes to see if you are all right.'

'[We] had lovely neighbours . . . no such thing as neighbours now . . . well you don't congregate same as like on bonfire night. In the old days all the neighbours used to be outside with chairs and what have you . . . having treacle toffee and roasted potatoes and all this lot, nobody cares about you now.'

'It was that nice on this estate. As I say, I was the first one in this house. When I moved in here it got full up this estate because it was that nice, well kept you know . . . I mean that . . . we all used to all be sat outside there with our sunshades and tables and you could leave them tables there all night and sunshades, go to bed, go out next morning and they'd still be there. Not now . . .'

(All quotes from Scharf *et al.* 2005: 20 and 24)

Isolation and loneliness

Wenger and her co-authors make a distinction between *social isolation*, which is an objective state defined as having minimal contact with other people, and *loneliness*, which refers to a subjective state of 'negative feelings associated with perceived social isolation, a lower level of contact than that desired or the absence of a specific desired companion' (Wenger *et al.* 1996). That reduction of isolation and loneliness should be a main aim of services is widely agreed.

Growing older often involves stressful life events such as bereavement, moving house and retirement. These can lead to greater isolation that in turn is associated with poorer health, a growing fear of crime, and insufficient income. More women than men experience loneliness because they frequently live longer than men and outlive partners, but men experience a greater intensity of loneliness than women. Wenger and colleagues point out that the principal criterion for isolation is living alone whereas in fact many older people, though living alone, do lead socially active lives and have close friendships that are more important than thinning family ties. Thus all those who are isolated do live alone, but the reverse is not true (Wenger *et al.* 1996).

While older people may turn to family for instrumental help, they are least likely to do this in times of loneliness. Loneliness is more closely associated with loss than with isolation. Both isolation and loneliness are associated with poor health and with diminishing contact with health professionals and use of medicines. They are also associated with admission to residential care, depression and poor recovery from strokes. Dying is both lonely and, for many, an isolated experience (Wenger *et al.* 1996).

OUTCOMES FOR OLDER PEOPLE

A number of outcomes for older adults using health and social care services have been developed since 1997 when the Department of Health commissioned extensive research and development projects. The most important of these, the OPUS project, (Older People's Utility Scale for Social Care), has identified six outcomes:

- personal comfort
- social participation and involvement
- food and nutrition
- safety
- control over daily living
- occupation (Netten *et al.* 2006).

Older people placed the greatest importance on personal comfort, followed by social participation and involvement, control over daily living and finally food and nutrition. But such preferences are shaped by individual factors. Age for example shapes preferences in that people over 85 were more concerned about food and nutrition and less concerned about social contact than were younger respondents. People who lived with others placed far greater importance on social participation and involvement than those who lived alone, while older people with disabilities saw food and nutrition as the highest priority (Henwood and Waddington 2002).

The green paper on adult services, *Independence, Well-being and Choice* (DOH 2005c), promotes similar outcomes: independence through choice and personal control, equal opportunity for work, participation in society without facing discriminatory hurdles, intentional or unintentional, improving health and quality of life, enabling people to make a positive contribution and have choice and control, ensuring freedom from discrimination or harassment, economic well-being and maintaining personal dignity.

Promoting the well-being of older people

Promoting the well-being of older people and its close relationships to neighbourhood has been closely explained in the Audit Commission's report *Older People – independence and well-being* (Audit Commission 2004; Carrier 2005). Based on work with focus groups convened by Age Concern, the report highlights what older people themselves regard as essential for their independence. This includes:

- neighbourhood
- housing
- social activities and social networks

- getting out and about
- income
- information
- health.

What older people regard as important is wider than services had previously acknow-ledged. Their well-being hinges on elements that most citizens of any age want: to participate, to be interdependent and be able to engage in reciprocal social relationships. They want to be seen as full citizens of their communities and not just as consumers of health services. They want to be able to create their own options and to be in full control of their lives.

To do this we need to invert the service triangle, placing the emphasis on community-based services that promote well-being for older people, with acute services as a smaller component (Local Government Association 2003; Carrier 2005; see Figure 7.2).

Dignity is highly valued by older people and should be deemed an outcome in its own right. Easily eroded, it is hard to shore up after it has been diminished. According to Woolhead and colleagues, dignity is constitutive of identity, autonomy and control. But they show how easily dignity of older people is jeopardised by a lack of community focus and the absence of structured choice within that community. They found it diminished by being patronised, excluded from decision making and being treated as an object. Ensuing lack of trust in society only increased older people's sense of physical risk and vulnerability. The evidence 'showed that person centred care for older people needs to be specifically related to communication, privacy, personal identity and feelings of vulnerability' (Woolhead *et al.* 2004).

NEIGHBOURHOOD-BASED SERVICES FOR OLDER PEOPLE

The white paper on health, *Our Health, Our Care, Our Say* (DoH 2006a), has emphasised the necessity of moving social services and health services to a preventive orientation and working for improvement in adults' well-being. It envisages new roles for social workers as navigators and brokers for local authority adult services, while relying on the voluntary and community sector not only to provide services but also to be advocates for individuals and innovative practice.

Such an orientation requires considerable changes. The trend in services for older people is to offer fewer services at higher cost. Disabled people discover this when crossing the age line – turning 65 – and suddenly find they are classified as 'older people' by social services departments with an accompanying lower level of service than they had previously received. For example, home care support plays a critical role in pre-serving independence. For every unit increase of home care the likelihood of remaining at home rose by 8 per cent (Davey *et al.* 2005). Yet Davey and her colleagues found that pressures on the home care services led to 'a bureaucratic, impersonal style of delivery which left little time for staff roles to focus on anything other than personal care, was risk averse and did not help in relation to improving wider outcomes' (Davey *et al.* 2005). They also considered how social care packages contributed to outcomes.

Support for older people today

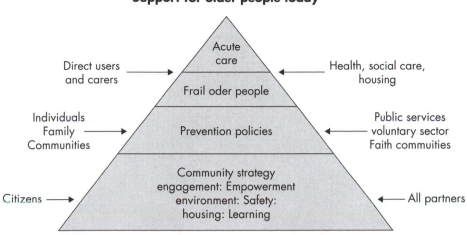

FIGURE 7.1 Inverting the triangle of care: support for older people today (LGA and ADSS 2003; Carrier 2005)

Support for older people tomorrow

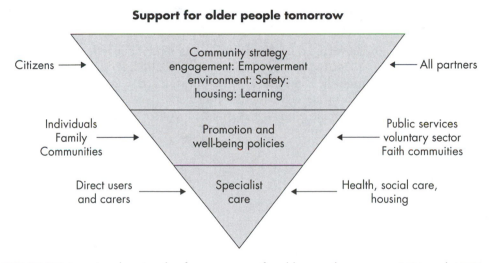

FIGURE 7.2 Inverting the triangle of care: support for older people tomorrow (LGA and ADSS 2003; Carrier 2005)

Whether high intensity home care (over ten hours per week), meals on wheels or day care (including lunch clubs), the most commonly reported outcome addressed by services packages was personal comfort, closely followed by cleanliness and comfort of accommodation. The outcomes least frequently addressed were occupation and social participation (Davey *et al.* 2005).

Effective day care services, home care and chiropody can all be said to support well-being, but independence requires more than that. Fear of crime, poor transport and inaccessible buildings also undermine independence and choice. All partners need to engage and enthuse over a shared vision – agree on priorities and what is meant

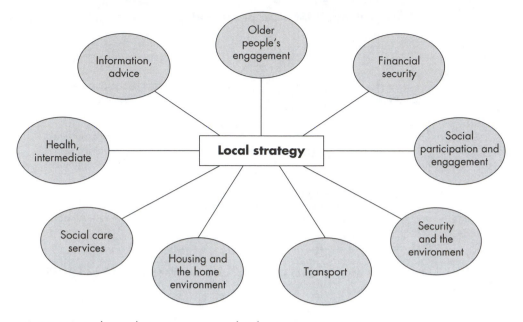

FIGURE 7.3 Making it happen; creating a local strategy (Carrier 2005)

by prevention – and then shape the local drive for enabling independence. The focus on risk needs to be broadened to include not just risks to health but other kinds of risks: risk of exclusion, of diminished status in society, of dispirited networks. There is still the powerful legacy of an earlier generation of policy and services rooted in the Poor Law's conception of pauperism, with its prescribed loss of social function and services through large institutional arrangements.

Prevention

Prevention in the context of adult services means taking action in the present to prevent the need for intensive or intrusive interventions in the future. In contrast to children's services, what is being 'prevented' is not the loss of developmental capacities early in the child's life course but a forestalling of the intrusiveness, loss of dignity and stripping of autonomy which accompany institutional intervention, for example enforced hospitalisation and entry into residential care with the consequent loss of network and onrush of social isolation.

   Independence for older people is achieved by building 'interdependence through networks and coalitions of individual, family, carers and community capacity' (Bremner 2005: 33). Preventive practice means tackling social exclusion and the stigma of ageism in order 'to build community capacity and to support communities of interest, as well as geographical communities to look after and manage their own affairs' (Bremner 2005: 33). By itself social care cannot address this scale of task but has to work with other elements of the local authority, all departments of which should be consulting community care user groups.

SHORING UP SUPPORT NETWORKS

Social networks can offer concrete forms of support, whether emotional ties or material aid such as contact, visits, errands or phone calls on behalf of an older person. Such networks are, however, subject to a range of variables – size, density, composition (in terms of roles, gender, age, material resources) and geographical spread of members. The capacity of networks relies on the strength and continuity of these personal ties – but also on the ideas and views that those in the network have about how much support should be offered and how much accepted, and the values and personality of the person at the centre.

Particular pressures have compelled government and practitioners to rely more on the social networks of older people as a source of long-term care. These include fiscal restraint and the cost of 'community' care, an ageing population and the wish to remain at home on the part of older people themselves. At the same time demographic and social changes have weakened the capacity of these support networks. More women working (and fewer seeing it as their job alone to care for an older person), fewer children, higher rates of divorce and greater geographical mobility have all made family networks more fragile (Keating *et al.* 2003).

The particular life course of the older individual also clearly affects network formation: people who are older, unmarried, childless and in poor health are the least likely to have robust support networks, with those 85 or older having much smaller networks than those who are younger. (Not surprisingly, unmarried older people will have invested more in non-family supportive relationships and so may have still robust networks.) For those over 85 the loss of same-generation relatives and friends and the tendency to put energy into only the closest relationships (Keating *et al.* 2003) can undermine what a support network is capable of achieving.

The difference between support networks and care networks

The size of a social network is not always a reliable predictor of support since any network may contain ties that have lost their friendship roles or have become impersonal. Support is unlikely to come from networks that have thinned in this way, but is more likely from those with continuing contact who form a subset within the larger network. Such a subset might include immediate family, relatives or particular neighbours. Networks of both family and friends have the widest capacity to perform tasks and give substantial amounts of support. This may include emotional support tasks such as providing social interaction, reassurance, validation, cheering up and monitoring as well as material support such as household jobs like preparing meals, cleaning, shopping for food, providing transport, bill paying and banking. But it is unwise for practitioners to make the assumption that older people who apparently have sufficient social ties will have the support they need. Support networks (with on average five to ten people) are smaller than the personal social networks (on average twelve to thirteen) from which they come and are usually found among long-standing kinship and friendship ties with high expectations to provide reciprocal support (van Tilburg 1998).

Care networks are even smaller than support networks (on average between three and five members) and the demands on them are correspondingly higher (although the terms are often used interchangeably). Older people with small support networks are very likely to have even smaller care networks, although in practice it is often difficult to discern the difference. 'Support' for a frail older person is in effect functional care-giving and should be designated care since it can exhaust the resources of the support network. Small as they are, networks perform different functions: adult children for example often maintain contact and provide some emotional and instrumental support, while siblings and friends provide mostly emotional support and companionship. Individual values and a sense of obligation play a powerful role in the kinds of support social networks are able to offer, as do gender relations and cultural attitudes within ethnic minorities and majorities and faith groups (Keating *et al.* 2003).

Support network	Levels and social context	Significance for practice
Locally integrated	Low contact May occur in context of mental illness Frail older person, living alone, withdraws from contact	• Where isolation occurs, usually results in shift to local self-contained network
Wider community focused	Low contact May occur in context of increasing frailty Local friendship network protects from isolation	• Where isolation occurs, usually results in shift to private restricted network
Local self-contained	High, well tolerated contact Associated with private lifestyle, self-sufficiency and living alone Exacerbated by failing health Living alone with low level of neighbour contacts	• Neighbour monitoring may help to avoid unrecognised crises • Good neighbour schemes likely to be well received • Home care at high levels of dependency
Local family dependent	Low contact Frail older person sees only carer Contact with local family usually precludes isolation	• Sitter service or day care may ameliorate situation for both older person and carer
Private restricted	High, may be well tolerated contact Exacerbated by failing health and restricted mobility Living alone with restricted contact with neighbours	• Neighbour may cooperate with services to provide monitoring • Good neighbour schemes can be offered but may be refused • Home care at high levels of dependency

FIGURE 7.4 Wenger's five types of support networks for older people (adapted from Wenger 1997)

Network mapping

Social work has long been aware of the power of networks, and in developing eco-maps and other tools has been far in advance of other caring professions in mapping specific networks in relation to the people they work with. Nevertheless, some of this work has been schematic and oversimplified both in relation to the standard graphical representations and the limited view of the social world that the older person lives in. Indeed, the graphical sophistication of current network mapping efforts has moved well beyond the old eco-map formats. For practitioners aiming to strengthen parts of a network it is important to configure what effect each element of the network will have on outcomes such as dignity, independence and participation. To achieve this, elements of networks such as brokering roles, network reach, boundary spanners and peripheral players need to be clearly identified along with the specific kind of social sustenance they provide (Krebs and Holley 2006).

Identifying the extent and capacities of support and care networks can only be done with a thorough knowledge of local resources, connections between community groups and the role of informal carers. The most effective way is to establish specifically who is part of the network and who thinks of themselves as part of the network and then ask what the capacity of these network members is to undertake the care tasks. Helpful here is Keating and colleagues' distinction between 'social', 'support' and 'caregiving' networks as discussed above. Transitions between the three reveal a pattern: as the function becomes more narrowly defined and more time consuming and even burdensome the networks contract as they proceed from one phase to the other. They move away from the 'dyadic' or intimate person model of informal care provision in which the model of informal care focuses on individual caregivers and recipients (Keating *et al.* 2003: 121) to become networks under great pressure, more prone to breakdown, tension and open conflict.

ACTIVITY 7.1: IDENTIFYING NETWORKS

Think of three older people you are working with. Into which category do their networks fall? What conclusions can you draw about the formation and maintenance of those networks? Are there ways that you can extend the reach and capacity of those networks?

CHOICE, PERSONALISATION AND THE LOCAL MARKET FOR SERVICES

Our Health, Our Care, Our Say (DoH 2006a) puts the user at the centre of a new system of obtaining care. It completes a revolution that was first suggested nearly twenty years ago in the Griffiths Report (Griffiths 1988), namely to separate completely the role of assessment and commissioning of services from that of service provision. Commissioners now act in an advocacy role responding directly to the user and being accountable to him or her. They must think more widely in terms of support and draw on a wider range of community services, not just health or social care. To respond to user need and preference it suggests creating independent advocates to help users make informed choices. The role involves service brokerage and navigating, assisting the older citizen in ways quite separate from the process of need assessment and service allocation.

'Choice' is difficult to exercise since it involves pulling triggers in systems which, though familiar to the practitioners, are quite unknown territory for users. Users are quite prepared to enter into choosing services and, moreover, prepared to spend their money in pursuit of those choices, but not where they are uncertain about what they are getting. Numerous obstacles remain to older citizens understanding the care system, primarily to do with values and culture of the systems they become enmeshed in. A basic feature of public sector care is that health care is generally free at point of use while social care levies a charge. While this is clear to practitioners it is not always so to users. The care management role remains shadowy, even confusing, and providing information on its own is not sufficient to overcome this. In any case user difficulties with the system are not to do with practicalities of care so much as with the emotional difficulties that follow in the wake of the disturbances to their known and scripted routines.

To remedy the situation, advocates have proposed walk-in community centres offering mental health advice and access to specialist services, more psychological treatment and wider user choice. The aim is to change the system previously geared to risk management and acute illness into one that meets the needs of people with long-term or more common mental health problems. Within such an arrangement 'access workers' would provide entry to the system rather than GPs. The centres would act as a base for health, social care and voluntary sectors, and provide information and support focusing on physical and mental health and well-being (IPPR 2005).

ACTIVITY 7.2: IS CHOICE EASY?

The practitioner might think for a moment about the range of new and critical choices that people have to make in their lives. Look over the following list: retirement plans, gas and electric suppliers, what kind of family to live in, dental plans, bank accounts, schools, colleges.

What kinds of information are needed to make an informed choice in each instance? In which of these choices are you actually a 'chooser', that is a person who thinks actively about the possibilities before making a decision based on what is important in your life and the short- and long-term consequences of that decision? In which are you a 'picker', that is one who grabs this or that option and hopes for the best? (See Schwartz 2004: 75).

Imagine then that you are 80 years old and have spent the previous two weeks in hospital recovering from a broken hip. You are offered several options within your intermediate care plan, including, if needed, a return to a different hospital than the one you have been in. What information would you need to either agree or alter this plan?

ACTIVITY 7.3: SOCIAL CARE ASSESSMENT AND DECISION MAKING

Funding for social care services has been described as a lottery and is viewed with perplexity by users. Research into assessment judgements has shown that social workers ration services more strictly than older people's self-assessments suggest they should be rationed.

Think back over some of the main points in this chapter and how assessments for social care of older people are conducted in your locality. Would older users underestimate their own need? Or is it the other way around and it is in fact the practitioners who would more closely ration care support? Are carers' groups well resourced? Are they able to make a compelling case for resources in public?

Individual budgets

The concept of individual budgets, also part of the government's programme for change in adult services, is intended to give older people discretionary control of the money the government has, in effect, set aside for their needs. Individual budgets represent a step beyond direct payments, which often involve the user in difficult and time-consuming matters of hiring what are in effect employees. This system had been taken up by only a very small proportion of older people in 2004, partly because individual assistance to help navigate the system was not in place.

With individual budgets the money must be used to meet needs that an assessment has defined. It channels funding either as cash for direct payment, services brokered by an adviser or services commissioned by the local authority. There is evidence that individual budgets have improved services and users' perception of services, in the main because they could calibrate the services they sought into a more direct relationship to how they viewed the quality of their life, particularly extending into cultural and what is, condescendingly called 'leisure pursuits' (IPPR 2005).

Sure Start in later life

Sure Starts for older people make an explicit link between outcomes and neighbourhood in the way Sure Start galvanised local communities to reshape children's services (Social Exclusion Unit 2006). It commits government policy to move beyond the basic standards of maintaining health and income to focus on the right of older people to participate in their communities and to engage throughout their lives in meaningful roles and relationships. Sure Start for older people says very clearly that this can only be done by building 'inclusive communities that meet local needs where the contribution of older people is key to their success' (SEU 2006: 8).

Sure Start in later life means providing a single gateway to services and opportunities to be engaged in the locality. But the extent of improved participation and improved well-being relies as much on what the neighbourhood and community have to offer as on the individual qualities of the older person. Individuals, families and communities (neighbours, GPs, pharmacists, shopkeepers) need to consider the extent and cause of social isolation in their areas and to act in concert to ensure that isolation is reduced. Leisure pursuits, adult learning and volunteering can all be drawn on to raise the level of engagement of older people in their community (SEU 2006: 12).

INTERMEDIATE CARE AND REHABILITATION

Part of the life course of older people in their neighbourhoods inevitably entails higher probabilities of frailty and of physiological or psychological impairment. Whereas pursuing outcomes for children should lead to them realising their full potential as independent young adults, working toward outcomes for older people means having support systems based on the principles of dignity, choice and autonomy in place in order to respond to increasing frailty and ill-health. In this linking of health and social care systems with neighbourhood resources, important steps forward have been taken since 2001.

Intermediate care

Intermediate care aims to overcome the frequently fractious relationship between social care and health care services in order to minimise hospitalisation or long-stay residential care and to provide a smooth transition for older people between hospital and home if necessary. It is targeted at people who would otherwise face unnecessarily prolonged stays in hospital or inappropriate admission to acute in-patient care, long-term residential care or long-term NHS in-patient care. Intermediate care provides a comprehensive assessment, resulting in a structured individual care plan, the end point of which typically is to enable the older person to live at home. This may involve physiotherapy, treatment or other opportunities for recovery in short-term settings such as a residential home or sheltered housing and is provided free for up to six weeks (Department of Health 2001). A short-term episode of care or rehabilitation avoids or reduces hospitalisation and maximises the capacity for independent living at home. The Community Care (Delayed Discharges) Act 2003, which established the outlines of intermediate care responses, allows local authorities to charge for community care services if they last longer than six weeks. However, they are not compelled to and some local authorities are more flexible on this deadline.

CASE STUDY 7.1: FOLLOWING A STROKE

A woman of 84 is in hospital following a stroke. She is about to be discharged but needs a high level of support that her daughter, age 40 and her only offspring, is willing to provide. However, if the daughter, who is a lone parent with a seven-year-old son, is to provide the intensive care for her mother for these first few weeks, she will need someone to take her son to and from school and to look after him for periods after school. It may be that this could be arranged informally through a friend but if she needs to pay a child minder (or a friend who cannot take unpaid leave from work) a direct payment to help pay for someone to take her son to school is possible. This would be part of the intermediate care package since it would avoid a longer stay in hospital or residential care. If the daughter needed additional equipment or services, for example a chair lift or transport for her mother, this could also be arranged.

Intermediate care aims to improve the efficiency and effectiveness of the health and social care system as a whole through more effective use of acute capacity and reduction in waiting times. To do this requires joined-up work across a number of settings – home, care home, day centre or sheltered housing – in which environments are 'more or less therapeutic' (Martin *et al.* 2005). Choosing the right place for intermediate care to occur is critical and should be linked to an ethos of successful ageing that promotes activity and self-sufficiency.

In one baseline study *before* the introduction of an intermediate care service Young and colleagues found that across two social services departments emergencies came in a range of guises: falls, incontinence, confusion and poor mobility. Without intermediate care outcomes were essentially grim. They found that 36 per cent of 823 patients followed for a 12-month period experienced a gradual decline in levels of independence over that period combined with a high degree of carer stress. Significantly, there was little use of standard rehabilitation services for any of the older people in this baseline study (Young *et al.* 2005). A subsequent study by the same team *after* intermediate care services had been put in place showed marked improvements in independence and levels of carer stress (Young *et al.* 2005).

Rehabilitative environments in the community

The rehabilitation of older people who have been hospitalised is a complex, context-related process, with powerful emotional and individual factors at work (Martin *et al.* 2005). There is a difference between curative and restorative environments and in the minds of users and practitioners they frequently produce different feelings and responses. Home is felt to be a place of security and autonomy in contrast to day centres, residential homes or hospitals. In that sense, home may be restorative in its effect but is a place where only modest levels of medical treatment can be provided. Hospital provides the reverse, and practitioners and family members anxious to reduce levels of physical risk to the older person may well see it as the preferable environment.

Martin and colleagues' research focused on two types of rehabilitative environment: the 'homely' and the 'institutional'. Unsurprisingly, the older people they interviewed saw the home as the ideal environment, which accords with intermediate care's emphasis on the home as the place where functional improvement and autonomy is typically optimised. But they also noted limits to what can be achieved in the home, that people needed 'to escape' and have the company provided at a day centre.

Gesler's notion of 'therapeutic landscape' is relevant here: emotions, social relations and practices are associated with different places (Gesler 1992). Gesler wrote that such a landscape is a 'constantly evolving process, moulded by the interplay, the negotiation between, physical, individual, and social factors. Thus, therapeutic landscape becomes a geographic metaphor for aiding in the understanding of how the healing process works itself out in places' (Gesler: 1992: 743).

Single assessment process

The single assessment process seeks to bring together a number of agencies behind a common approach to assessment of older people and indeed in relation to other adults with mental health needs. There are three elements to the single assessment process recently developed for older people who wish to use health or social care services:

- it is centred on the older person
- it offers a common, standardised format for all services provided to the older person
- it is oriented towards delivering specified outcomes for that person.

To improve outcomes both for individuals and across an entire community the assessor must be able to provide the appropriate planning and services to enhance dignity, autonomy and social participation. While the process does not stipulate specific assessment tools, the research associated with outcomes for social care showed significant confusion over the process as a whole, particularly in relation to carers. For example, over half of all carers who had been assessed were unaware that any assessment had taken place. Further, there was poor consultation over interview arrangements, difficulties in completing the self-assessment forms, and a presumption that carers would simply carry on caring. Over half the carers did not receive any written follow-up to assessment so that they were not informed of decisions arising from the assessment (Henwood and Waddington 2002). A significant proportion of older people and their carers could remember little or nothing of their contact with social workers or what had happened (Levin and Illiffe 2004). Yet the same body of research showed that good practice in assessment is relatively easy to achieve if:

- the assessment process is made explicit
- carers are given adequate time and information to prepare for assessment interviews
- mutual arrangements for assessment are discussed
- opportunity is given for informed choice concerning privacy.

BOX 7.2: SINGLE ASSESSMENT PROCESS

The National Service Framework for Older People promotes the single assessment process that covers primary care trusts and general practice, community nursing, social care and specialist medical services. It also establishes integrated arrangements for commissioning and provision for services. New approaches include the development of integrated primary care and social services trusts.

The single national assessment framework seeks to achieve convergence of local assessment procedures with outputs and outcomes over time. Local agencies are required to demonstrate that their approach to assessment complies with the National Service Framework for Older People and government guidance. The purpose of the single assessment process is to ensure that older people receive appropriate, effective and timely responses to their health and social care needs, and that professional resources are used effectively.

- Age, of itself, should not determine how services are accessed or provided.
- Access to services should be via assessment that is coordinated and straightforward, with duplication kept to a minimum.
- Information sharing between professionals, where confidentiality is respected, can be crucial for effective person-centred care.
- Where an older person requires the help of more than one agency, agencies should coordinate service delivery in the best interests of the older person.
- Promoting health and well-being is as important as reacting and responding to needs as and when they arise.
- The potential for rehabilitation should be explored at assessment and subsequently kept under review.

Local implementation should be based on the geographical areas used for implementing the National Service Framework for Older People as a whole, for example the area covered by the local strategic partnerships. Where there are overlapping boundaries and impending changes to boundaries, local agencies should agree solutions that put the interests of service users first.

Agencies should reach an understanding of how medical diagnosis fits in the single assessment process. Medical diagnosis is the identification of a specific health condition, how it arose and its likely course. As such, medical diagnosis can be seen as distinct from the assessment of wider health and social care needs. However, because specific health impairments such as stroke or a fractured neck or femur are interlinked with social, physical and mental health needs, it makes separation of diagnosis and assessment unhelpful in practice.

(Adapted from DoH 2006 and DoH 2001)

THE SEAMLESS PATHWAY

Overall, the strategy around integrated care is designed to establish effective joint working between all practitioners involved in delivering care – not just on the health side (trusts and primary care trusts) but also social care agencies and voluntary and community organisations. The intention is to create the 'seamless pathway' through the health and social care system, offering a personalised care plan for those most at risk and reducing the numbers using acute beds, enabling a greater number of people over 65 to live at home. There are problems. Many emergency admissions have by-passed the GPs and primary care trusts. Chronic alcoholics, who make up a large sector of potential users, are difficult to work with. At the time of writing there are possible difficulties particularly over the role of community matron, who will act as case manager and perhaps have the power to withdraw from contracts and services from community providers and social care services. Lack of experience in case management in for example charging or commissioning services may further impede the seamless delivery (Hudson 2005).

Well-integrated teams do point the way forward. Such a team would include practitioners from housing, nursing, and social care but may also include personnel from mental health services for older people, occupational therapy, learning difficulties and acute services. There are, as Hudson reminds us, two models for integration. One is based on centralisation and specialistion and the other on localisation. It is quite possible to adopt the rhetoric of the second in order to cover the activities of the first, particularly when government prioritises choice and competition over collaboration.

CASE STUDY 7.2: PATHWAY TEAMS IN SEDGEFIELD

There are five integrated 'pathway' teams in Sedgefield, County Durham. Each brings together practitioners from different services: housing, nursing, social care, occupational therapy and mental health services. Team members enjoy a parity of esteem, that is to say there is no perceived difference in the status or importance of one team member compared to another. The teams have worked hard to transfer the sense of loyalty away from the earlier professional attachments to the new teams. The teams' effectiveness is based on the familiarity with each other's roles and responsibilities, which enables decisions to be made quickly. This flexibility and creativity around longstanding professional boundaries have enabled the teams to find innovative solutions to old problems of coordination. A network of middle managers from across the services designed the structure of the teams while kindred colleagues who supported the initiative were left to work out the operational and practice implications such as identifying staff with the necessary skills to join the teams. A partnership board, made up of users and representatives from the contributing services, defines the issues and sets the strategy for the pathway teams.

(Adapted from Hudson 2006)

COLLABORATION BETWEEN HEALTH AND SOCIAL CARE

The central collaborative element in delivering joined-up services for older people in neighbourhoods and communities is between health and social care. Since 1997 a steady stream of legislation, guidance and funding for special initiatives has encouraged partnership across that divide – referred to, with some reason, as 'the Berlin Wall': immovable, implacable, but ultimately to be torn down. The Health Act 1999 and the NHS Plan (DOH 2000) offer incentives to local councils and health authorities to exercise powers for joint working. There is a duty to form partnerships through pooled budgets, lead commissioning and integrated provision. The difficulty is that despite the prodding of central government, the real nature of what collaboration entails on the ground has not always been addressed.

Although the expectation of collaboration is high, health and social care do not easily combine and indeed have many elements in opposition. Far from differences being eased, it is clear that past divisions have not been wholly overcome. Professional cultures are still very different with each wanting the other to change its way of working more in line with its own. Huntington's research twenty years ago underscored the distinct occupational cultures and power differences between social workers (of all varieties) and general practitioners in the 1980s (Huntington 1981). She described this relationship as one of 'action versus holding orientation'. 'The medical training', she wrote, 'focuses on swift decision making to enable competent handling of emergency situations whereas social workers are taught that better decisions are made if a situation is contained until the opinions of all concerned are clarified' (Huntington 1981 cited in Kharicha et al. 2005: 404). Huntington also noted that differences in status, authority and prestige, knowledge and language acted as barriers to successful collaboration.

Twenty years later Kharicha and colleagues noted that, far from overcoming these barriers:

> the exact opposite has occurred, with a multitude of innovative pilot projects that never became mainstream forms of provision even in areas where joint administrative structures might have facilitated this, for example Northern Ireland so that debates about the merits of GP attachment of social workers still continue.
>
> (Kharicha et al. 2005: 400)

Understanding each other's professional orientation and in particular 'the clinical pole' and 'the social pole' within the health services and social work services respectively is crucial to effective work. One approach to foster joint working is 'co-location' – placing social workers and health staff in the same office. The thinking is that this would increase face-to-face contact and multi-disciplinary meetings and therefore improve collaboration (Kharicha et al. 2005: 401). While it improves collaboration on a day-to-day basis, social workers expressed a need for more formal contact with their health and social care colleagues in the form of regular, planned, multi-disciplinary meetings between frontline and managerial staff. They also sought the co-location of social and primary care staff who were absent.

As a learning environment and source of creativity, however, co-location proved a double-edged sword. Social workers felt it did *not* encourage health colleagues to understand the role of social workers but rather was a resource to buttress the essential health-oriented mission of the team. Social workers felt isolated by the dominant assumption that their resources and capabilities were routinely available. They would have preferred a system in which health practitioners made formal requests for the resources at their command. Researchers have concluded that co-location 'generated high expectations of working relations with health colleagues which could not always be met outside of that setting' (Kharicha et al. 2005: 402). There was also evidence of concern that service thresholds may change or be absorbed into multi-disciplinary practice teams and that practitioners would have difficulty in keeping to social work priorities and eligibility and risk criteria. Social workers in turn deployed avoidance strategies for resolving differences of opinion. These included:

- risk minimisation and pinpointing who takes responsibility
- conceding on policy
- accepting pragmatic solutions
- using nurses as mediators
- resorting to hierarchical authority (Kharicha *et al.* 2005: 403).

Part of the problem lies in the massive extension of activity that occurs under the health banner. Programmes aimed at behaviour change, once the preserve of psychologists, counsellors and social workers, are now enthusiastically taken up by nursing staff, who may be better trained in brief solution therapy than social workers from whose discipline it originally emerged. Nurses also routinely make assessments of families' capacity to care (Crist 2005). Here the distinction between health and social care is gone – evaporated within the new concept of 'family care' which the authors of the study deploy. Eco-maps, which social workers have used routinely for thirty years, have recently been taken up by nursing, which thinks of them as a new discovery (see for example Ray and Street 2005). In short, what were, in the hands of social workers, tools for understanding the complexities of social environments in a radically unequal society are, for nursing, methods for extending clinical influence and a clinical perspective.

In contemporary adult services the danger is that social care becomes a junior partner compelled to collaborate within a framework in which it is relatively powerless. The cuts in NHS funding in mid-2006 that led almost immediately to cuts in social care provided by local authorities are a telling example of a wider problem. The future may see the relegation of 'the social', in emerging care terminology, which will hold not only a narrow view of citizen autonomy but also be an expression of professional competence unbound.

KEY POINTS

☐ Older people want to participate in their neighbourhoods and communities; in this they are like any other citizen who wants to be involved in reciprocal relationships.

☐ Services for older people are being restructured to help older people achieve these outcomes and attain well-being.

☐ Emphasis on social networks points to the importance of neighbourhood and of responsive local services.

☐ The emphasis is on choice and control and above all recognising that well-being of older people relies on their being strongly connected to their neighbourhood in a reciprocal relationship, both contributing to and drawing on local supports.

☐ Collaboration with health services, though not without difficulties, is key to any effective joined-up provision: the single assessment process, intermediate care pathways and Sure Start in later life all require close engagement with the local community.

CHAPTER 8

BRINGING COMMUNITIES TOGETHER: OVERCOMING FAITH AND ETHNIC DIVIDES

OBJECTIVES

By the end of this chapter you should:

▪ Understand the role of faith in defining and overcoming ethnic difference and community divides

▪ Understand how 'us' and 'them' thinking becomes established in a locality

▪ Understand central government policy on community cohesion

▪ Be familiar with mediation skills and the role that social work can play in developing a sense of commonality in localities.

This chapter considers some of the factors that appear to cause division and conflict in Britain's cities and towns. It lays out the background that gave rise to the government's policies on community cohesion from 2001 and the substance of that policy. It also examines the renewed importance of culture and religion within communities and explains how practitioners, building on their long-held commitment to anti-racist and anti-oppressive practice, can use tools of mediation and dialogue to defuse local conflict.

FRACTURED COMMUNITIES?

Following the civil disturbances in some northern cities in the summer of 2001 between white and Asian young men, the police and far right groups, the government moved swiftly to tackle what it saw as communities fractured by ethnic and faith divides. The series of reports that followed the disorders, including the Cantle Report (Home Office 2001) and the Ousley Report (Ousley 2001), highlighted the lack of integration between different 'communities' in those cities and by extension in many of the major cities of Britain, whether or not they had experienced any open conflict.

What seems to have caught government by surprise was the extent of the gulf between different ethnic and religious communities. While it had been established that American patterns of segregation and racialised ghettos had *not* developed in the UK (Peach 1996), nevertheless the degree of residential separation and its impact on identity and opportunity was far stronger than previously assumed. The question has been posed with new urgency and the answers have been anxious and provisional. In 2005 the former head of the Commission for Racial Equality, Lord Ousley, and its current chairman, Trevor Phillips, both warned that continuing segregation, particularly of Asian neighbourhoods, pointed towards fully fledged ghettos. Phillips noted the coming of 'a New Orleans style Britain of passively coexisting ethnic and religious communities, eyeing each other over the fences of our differences' (quoted in Gilan 2005).

BOX 8.1: THE CANTLE REPORT SUMMARISES ITS FINDINGS

Whilst the physical segregation of housing estates and inner city areas came as no surprise, the team was particularly struck by the depth of polarisation of our towns and cities. The extent to which these physical divisions were compounded by so many other aspects of our daily lives was very evident. Separate educational arrangements, community and voluntary bodies, employment, place of worship, language, social and cultural networks mean that many communities operate on the basis of a series of parallel lives. These lives often do not seem to touch at any point, let alone overlap and promote any meaningful interchanges.

(Home Office 2001: 9)

The geographical concentration of ethnic minorities in urban neighbourhoods does indeed have an impact on job prospects, training and educational attainment and labour market participation. Clark and Drinkwater (2002), using data from the 1991 census, established that although the ethnic minority population of three million comprised 6 per cent of the total population in England and Wales, 31 per cent lived in wards where minorities accounted for over 50 per cent of the population, and the top 19 per cent of wards defined by ethnic minority density contained around 64 per cent of all minority residents in the country. Their investigation showed conclusively that the existence of such enclaves of ethnically concentrated neighbourhoods impacts upon the opportunities and constraints facing residents of such areas: variation in employment outcomes, lower incidence of self-employment (contradicting the conventional wisdom of ethnic entrepreneurship) and higher rates of unemployment. Higher levels of deprivation meant lower consumer activity and a reduced set of economic opportunities and pushed white workers to migrate to the suburbs following the outward movement of jobs, further highlighting the inability of minorities to do so. To an extent, public services, particularly housing and education, have reinforced this pattern (Clark and Drinkwater 2002).

COMMUNITY COHESION POLICIES

Government recognised that the disturbances and underlying conflict severely tested its concepts of multiculturalism and multicultural citizenship. From 2001 it sought to break down the barriers between culturally and physically segregated populations whether black, Asian or white through a sustained policy of 'community cohesion'. This policy broadly aimed to promote common understanding and dialogue across 'communities within communities' at the same time as emphasising the common values that all citizens and people resident in Britain should share.

While the policy was broadly developed within a number of pathfinders in 2001, it soon acquired national scope. The National Action Plan on Social Inclusion defined community cohesion as a central aspect of its wider social inclusion agenda, suggesting that areas most at risk of community tensions are also those with high levels of social exclusion (Department of Work and Pensions 2003). The sources of conflict as viewed by government (Home Office 2001; Ousley 2001) stem from several factors:

- communities living in isolation from one another, arising from housing segregation, whether the housing is owner-occupied a social housing
- lack of common leisure, recreational, sporting and cultural activities
- poor joint working between community, faith and business leaders
- resentment over public monies funding projects in some neighbourhoods but not others
- schools dominated by a single culture
- provocative racist attacks.

BOX 8.2:   WHAT IS A 'COHESIVE' COMMUNITY?

A cohesive community is one where:

- a common vision and sense of belonging prevails
- the diversity of people's different backgrounds and circumstances is appreciated and positively valued
- similar life opportunities are provided for all, regardless of background
- strong and positive relationships are developed between people from different backgrounds and circumstances in the workplace, in the school and in neighbourhoods.

(Local Government Association 2004)

Promoting cohesion in the government's perspective means addressing those divisions, removing barriers and encouraging positive interaction between groups. The intention of government is to embed tackling the concerns about segregation and community conflict into its regeneration and neighbourhood renewal policies. This will require all services to tackle segregation and ethnic enclaves by broadening their practice on social inclusion. In this effort, education, planning, economic development and social care have distinct contributions to make. The Neighbourhood Renewal Unit is clear that the body of knowledge and skills used to help people, groups or communities find consensual strategies and common ground on which they can live and work together is applicable across much of the work of community development, community health and education, youth work, social work, anti-racism, equal opportunity and equality work (NRU 2005). Local authorities have been asked to prepare community cohesion plans as part of their community strategy in order to promote cross-cultural contact and foster mutual understanding and respect.

Broadly, government policy aims to achieve the following through its community cohesion policies:

- reinforce ideas of common citizenship
- compel political parties and local services to engage in dialogue and give strong leadership
- institute programmes to promote contact between faiths and ethnic groups
- secure the participation of young people in the locality
- end monoculture schools
- develop mixed (integrated) housing
- pursue equal access to employment locally
- have trained personnel across services and in the community in conflict resolution (Home Office 2005).

The potential for success of this policy rests on the assumption that common principles and shared values can ultimately be found in a multi-ethnic and multi-faith society. Yet in diverse communities this is by no means certain and in any case there are no short cuts. As Madeleine Bunting has written:

> A comfortable multicultural society is . . . made on the street, in the school – in the myriads of relationships of friends, neighbours and colleagues. That's where new patterns of accommodation to bridge cultural differences are forged; that's where minds change, prejudices shift and alienation is eased.
> (Bunting 2006)

Existing community cohesion policy also de-emphasises deprivation and socio-economic marginalisation in favour of focusing on inter-community relationships, and thus says little directly about the forces behind this marginalisation (McGhee 2003). Finally, government policy seems to expect community leaders to shoulder near-impossible responsibilities. For example, in effect it is saying to Muslim communities, 'Islamic extremism is your problem; sort out your co-religionists, calm them down (and anything you can do to get their boys to study harder and their wives to go to work will be welcome)' (Bunting 2006).

Pursuing cohesion has significantly changed the orientation of the government's anti-racist strategies (Worley 2005). While continuing to promote respect for all cultures it now places far more emphasis on social integration and shared values and deracialises local politics, playing down racism as a potent element in community discourses. The strong commitments to tackling institutional racism embodied in the Stephen Lawrence report (Macpherson 1999) and the Race Relations (Amendment) Act of 2000 have been downgraded.

There is also a perceptible shift in government policy as to what constitutes citizenship. Multicultural definitions of citizenship recognised that different groups have different values, interest and needs and should enjoy rights of 'recognition' and respect. While there were problems with this approach, namely that it often ignored differences *within* particular cultures and overlooked the fluidity of boundaries between ethnic groups including white British, it nevertheless provided a framework of rights as part of a mosaic of cultures. Now members of ethnic minorities (remembering of course that in many urban areas they are majorities) are facing a narrower definition of citizenship and being asked to adopt a set of shared national values. The hope is to build communities where people feel confident not only that they belong but that they can mix and interact with others, particularly people from different racial backgrounds or people from different faiths (Local Government Association 2004). The difficulty is that the 'shared national values' may largely derive from a received idea of 'national heritage' formed at a time before Britain became a place of cultural diversity.

ACTIVITY 8.1: A TEST FOR CITIZENSHIP?

Read the following text from a recent Home Office report on strengthening society.

> For those settling in Britain, the Government has a clear expectation that they will integrate into our society and economy because all the evidence indicates that this benefits them and the country as a whole. . . . We consider that it is important for all citizens to have a sense of inclusive British identity. This does not mean that people need to choose between Britishness and other cultural identities, nor should they sacrifice their particular lifestyles, customs and beliefs. They should be proud of both.
> (*Improving Opportunity, Strengthening Society*, Home Office 2005: 45)

With a small group of colleagues, discuss the following questions related to the text:

Is there such a thing as 'Britishness'? If so, how is it defined?

Should all new arrivals to Britain learn the English language?

Should there be basic tests for gaining UK citizenship?

How do community cohesion policies differ from the old and now discredited notion of 'assimilation', that all cultures should blend in with that of the wider society?

THE ANTI-RACIST HERITAGE OF SOCIAL WORK

To its great credit, social work was among the first profession to require an anti-racist perspective and anti-oppressive practice as one of its principle objectives for all practitioners (Central Council for Education and Training in Social Work (CCETSW) 1991). It developed the competencies, the values, the commitment and ethos to challenge racist practices wherever they were encountered – be it within their own or other agencies, amongst professionals, in the local media or in community meetings. The approach was rigorous, not confined to interpersonal transactions but willing to tackle wider structural features (such as institutional racism) as well as prevailing stereotypes and everyday oppressive language. The size and scale of that commitment should be acknowledged, for it demonstrated what practitioners could professionally commit themselves to in pursuing social change.

It is worth recalling, however briefly, the extent of that professional commitment to tackling racism. Much of it lay in recognising the scale of racism and realising how far short its own services fell in reversing racism. Whether meeting the needs of Asian elders, tackling the disproportionate number of young black men in the criminal justice system, highlighting the racialised system of mental health diagnoses or the problems besetting black children in care, the profession did systematically attempt to resolve its own shortcomings. At another level it promoted a more sophisticated view of what racism entailed: the understanding that assimilation and 'colour blind' perspectives inherently perpetuated race-based oppression. It had developed a critique of institutional racism well before the Macpherson report into the murder of Stephen Lawrence (Macpherson 1999). The important conclusion for our purpose here is that this was a practice that made no distinction between the various sectors of the ecological model. Rather it ranged across the levels of individual, family, neighbourhood and community in order to tackle stereotypes, intervene in public discussion and present challenging arguments within local and national media.

The transition of this commitment, however, into the twenty-first century world, a world more fractured by faith, has not been smooth, and professional commitments to newer forms of anti-oppressive practice appear more dilute. Although the same structurally oppressive and racist factors are in place, namely that race, minority ethnicity and some faiths are strongly associated with disadvantage, social and economic status and geographical concentration, the mix of these factors appears to be regarded more tentatively and with greater uncertainty. Thus far social work has been more reticent in articulating a position as clear and as committed as it did in the earlier struggles against racism.

The remainder of this chapter looks at how practitioners might better understand this more fractured, postmodern world and how it might rework its mission to take on board tasks that are in many ways parallel to the anti-racist struggle of the 1980s and 1990s. Key to this understanding is a deeper appreciation of the significant role that culture and values increasingly play in people's lives, especially, in some communities, religious values, and how skills in mediation and conflict resolution could defuse some of the worst divisions in the localities in which they work.

THE RENEWED IMPORTANCE OF CULTURE AND RELIGION

We are living in a period of revival of faith in which cultural 'values' are invoked more readily to explain the loss of social cohesion. Where once socio-economic factors alone were regarded as the primary source of social tensions, and later race and ethnic differences, now faith has also been added to the account. To some extent, social work has shied away from considering these kinds of cultural explanations of social conflict partly because they may appear to blame the victim and partly because it has at best felt awkward in its relationship to religion and at worst openly antagonistic to many tenets of many faiths, particularly in relation to dogma concerning women and sexual orientation.

Moreover, for much of the second half of the twentieth century it was assumed that as societies grew richer and more modern they would become more secular. This secularisation thesis broadly forecast that as people became better educated, religious tenets would lose their dominant place in shaping different cultures. Moreover, as communications technology improved, there would be greater cooperation and understanding. As voters became more educated, they would become more ecumenical and independent-minded. In that sense secularisation meant that there was little need for any hard thinking on the role of religion in society.

However, in the last twenty years, as people have been empowered by greater wealth and education, cultural differences have become more pronounced, not less, as different groups pursue different visions of the good life, and react strongly to attacks on their cultural dignity. As adjustments are made to the secularisation thesis (at least in the short term) a different insight into politics also emerges: the notion that groups will pursue their interests within a pluralist, democratic framework – accepting the democratic rules and the inevitable compromises that goes with it – is no longer so clear cut.

To explain this phenomenon sociologists such as Anthony Giddens (Giddens 1991), Zygmunt Bauman (Bauman 2001) and Ulrich Beck (Beck 1992) among others argue that individuals living in the twenty-first century have to choose among an array of competing demands and values as the demands from their social and working life are constantly changing under constraint from the global market world order. The individual must negotiate a constantly changing environment just to remain employable or to stay in relationships. This always provisional knowledge produces a contemporary form of existential anxiety, which becomes particularly acute when individuals find themselves facing phenomena that that knowledge cannot explain.

Religious knowledge and experience does provide the moral resources to tackle such anxiety (Henery 2003; Giddens 1991). It faces death head on, whereas 'the abstract system of modernity makes death a matter of problems about which something can be done – in relation to this or that illness . . . or threat to health. Modernity can only deal with what can be adapted and manipulated' (Henery 2003: 1107).

BOX 8.3:   SOCIAL CAPITAL, FAITH AND COMMUNITY

Broadly defined, 'social capital' represents the collective efficacy stored in the social relations, value norms and sense of trust embedded in the social networks of a community. Amid speculation that social capital is in decline, religious involvement and religious institutions have been identified as important sources and carriers of social capital. Indeed, one important authority has deemed faith communities as 'the single most important repository of social capital in America' (Putnam 2000: 66).

A number of investigations offer support for the contention that faith institutions generate social capital in the localities where they are situated. Furbey and colleagues (Furbey *et al.* 2006) for example found that faith offers institutional means through which people of different religions (or none) are able to come together in ways that are not always recognised. Religious buildings can be significant places where local people can cross boundaries, meet others, share activities and build trust. Faith communities can facilitate making links across a locality by developing new forms of association, bringing a spirit of trust to shared community initiatives and motivating particular approaches to social justice and human need. They have distinctive priorities, working styles and commitments to particular neighbourhoods. Farnell and colleagues reached similar conclusions in their extensive investigation of faith communities in neighbourhood regeneration programmes (Farnell *et al.* 2003). Religious affiliation has also been linked to higher levels of formal volunteering, learning civic skills, informal caregiving, and participation in small support groups. Park and Smith (2000), for example, found that religiosity positively influences levels of volunteering in the localised community because participation in the religious sphere brings with it the development of skills and attitudes reflective of helping others.

Robert Wuthnow (2002) found a positive correlation between membership of a faith organisation and 'bridging' social capital, which is all the more difficult to sustain because it requires that people look beyond their immediate social circles and depends on institutions being capable of and wanting to nurture cooperation among heterogeneous groups. Pierson and Gill (2005) also looked closely at the relationship between community development and faith institutions in a low-income district of a major city in the West Midlands. They found that:

- The extent of contribution that faith institutions make to their local communities varies, depending on how the local political culture shapes local ideas of identity, especially as defined by race and religion.
- Subordinate groups have different spaces in which to be political – formal institutions may only constitute a small proportion of social interaction; faith institutions can offer both formal and informal political 'space'.
- 'Segmented' assimilation of second- and third-generation Muslims means that mosques offer tight social networks, precise values and strong rules of behaviour for some but not all local residents.
- There are common barriers in all faiths to the inclusion of gays and lesbians in their faith institutions.
- There is a tension between spiritual and community matters. As one leader involved in

community cohesion efforts said: 'those of us who are involved with community cohesion have got to keep in contact with our religious roots, without our religious training we're not going to be any use to the people'.

- Many professionals working in the city generally ignored the shifting dynamics of religiously inspired social network behaviour and how that behaviour fits within a broader pattern of identity formation for individuals and faith collectives.

Working with faith communities

Working with people of faith both within faith communities and across religious divides presents extraordinary challenges to practitioners. For example they may have their own religious beliefs which contradict professional ethical positions in relation to end of life decisions, abortion, or sexual orientation. But the greater challenge is to better understand the sense of what faith means to adherents, to develop effective links with local faith institutions and to define the approaches that work in bringing communities divided by faith together.

The recent focus on spirituality has proved an entry point for social work to take stock of its secular orientation and to move the profession as a whole toward more explicit regard for the spiritual dimension and beliefs of users, as part of understanding the whole person, whatever practitioners' own beliefs and experiences may be.

Spirituality has been defined as a way of living that gives deliberate consideration to the transcendent dimension of human experience (Banja 1995, cited in Ai 2002). Addressing the spiritual needs of local residents and service users has become more urgent given the pace of socio-cultural change and dislocation experienced by many in the urban communities of advanced industrial countries such as Britain. Spirituality allows practitioners to respond to ultimate questions concerning the meaning and purpose of life without necessarily having to involve themselves in the organised doctrine and practices of particular faiths (Ai 2002). The emphasis on spirituality particularly in work with children, older people and adults with mental health problems has opened the profession toward working with people of faith more sympathetically. In a sense, then, religion is subsumed under this older, wider notion of human spiritual need.

There are ambiguous consequences for practitioners however in the concept of spirituality, particularly for those engaging in community practice. It constructs religious choice as an element of lifestyle in which the individual acquires a sense of achievement and relief from anxiety but does not explore religion as an institutional resource that often has strong commitments to achieving social justice and tackling poverty in local communities. Henery (2003) argues that whereas religion presents a challenge to consumer capitalism because it does not emphasise a lifestyle of product acquisition, spirituality does not. It finds its place alongside popular self-help books and through this popular literature renders religion as a resource for lifestyle management, presented as highly individualistic and often based on uniquely personal experiences. 'It does this homeopathically', Henery argues in a telling phrase, 'by giving us a small enough dose of the bug we are inoculated against the disease [of religion]' (Henery 2003: 1108). The spirituality project becomes a way of containing religion; the discussions it initiates are those in which customs, institutions and liturgy are avoided while there is an emphasis on 'personal journey', self-expression and individual experience.

Despite the strength of Henery's criticism it may be that within a relatively secular and multicultural environment matters of belief have to be approached in general as a human phenomenon, in which social workers recognise spiritual understanding as important for some users and that they can assist in the development of personal beliefs, acknowledge experiences of awe and feelings of transcendence (Kibble *et al.* 2001).

However social workers in community practice need to go beyond this. In communities and neighbourhoods where the majority of people adhere strongly to specific beliefs faith institutions have considerable resources to bolster communities, particularly in low income neighbourhoods where other institutions have frayed or disappeared altogether. In addition there are elements of belief in all the major faiths that promote social justice, tackle poverty and exclusion and join with other institutions in renewing the social fabric (Noor 2000; Shupe and Misztal 1998; Williams 2005).

BOX 8.4: GOOD PRACTICE WHEN ENGAGING FATIH COMMUNITIES

- Before engaging in discussions with those from faith groups, find out about their beliefs. However do not let lack of knowledge prevent talking to people. An open, positive approach usually produces a positive response.
- Be aware of regular days and times of worship of different faith groups and organize meetings and events accordingly.
- Be sensitive in the choice of venue and the types of food provided.
- Establish particular structures, such as a multi-faith forum that may assist faith communities in expressing their views.
- Think carefully as to how appointment of representatives of particular faiths to partnership boards will be viewed by people of other faiths or from different traditions within the same faith.

(Adapted from Ahmed 2000)

CASE STUDY 8.1: CHILDREN AND RELIGIOUS FAITH

Smith and Khanom (2005) have developed a useful typology based on their research with over 100 children aged between 9 and 11:

- 'highly observant' – heavily involved in the practices and institutions of their faith and strongly committed to the values they are taught

- 'observant' – their faith is a significant and regular part of their lives
- 'occasionally participating' – only participate infrequently and are unlikely to be well grounded in their faith and its practices
- 'implicit individual faith' – have moved beyond the specific practices of their faith and while they may belong to specific religious institutions that is not essential to how they understand what faith is
- 'not religious' – have little interest in or understanding of their religion or of religion in general apart from what they have learned in school.

These different categories of experiences provide practitioners with indicators for understanding children's behaviour in relation to other children of other faiths both in school and outside. As Smith and Khanom explain:

> The research points to growing evidence that religious difference is becoming a marker for hostility between groups, and that children are being actively discouraged by adults from mixing across religions where there are significant levels of racism and intolerance evident in wider society.
>
> (Smith and Khanom 2005: 4)

The more observant children spent more time on their faith, which impacted on their relationships out of school – the more devout the child, the less interaction with other children from outside the faith (than less devout children) (Smith and Khanom 2005: 4). 'Many of the friendship circles were religiously and ethnically homogenous' they noted.

Another finding revealed that children recognise local places of worship – but very few have visited other places than their own. On no occasion did the schools involved organise visits to different places of worship, suggesting that they are not seen as a local resource for the whole community.

UNDERSTANDING THE EXPERIENCE OF NEW ARRIVALS TO SETTLED COMMUNITIES

Recent work on what it is like to uproot from a home country and move to another has expanded our understanding of what is involved in the settling-in process. Werbner (2005) has argued that people newly arrived in another country rely on their distinctive culture that sets themselves apart from host societies in order to sink roots in their new country. They strive to retain a morally compelling vision that provides a source of relatedness, agency and power in a daunting environment. Her investigation of Britain in the 1960s shows how Pakistani communities developed their own cultural institutions, not as a source of nostalgia but as necessary bulwarks for the long haul. The early arrivals were mostly young men in the 1950s and 1960s who instituted a system of dyadic, interest-free loans among themselves to help buy property, marry or bring their families over. The loans provided a way of establishing friendship but also followed Punjabi rules and expectations concerning the purposes of such loans, underpinning verbal agreements and extending times for repayment. As families began arriving in Britain to join these men, women struggled to recapture their control over another crucial area of social exchange: the Punjabi gift economy, *lena dena*, or giving and taking, instituting for instance communal neighbourhood readings of the Koran followed by a food offering (Werbner 2005).

The immigrant's ethnicity, culture and ancestry provide a variable source of strength. There are those who will be able to use their networks and resources of solidarity to improve themselves socially and economically. But there are also those whose ethnicity will be viewed antagonistically by the settled community, placing them at risk of joining the dispossessed and excluded, compounding the inequality and despair in inner cities where they are compelled to settle (Portes 2003:43).

This affords the second generation of immigrant families both opportunities and dangers. Role reversal may happen in relation to their parents – when children's acculturation moves so far ahead of their parents that information on which to base key family decisions becomes dependent on children's knowledge – they speak the language and are more familiar with the host culture. Yet disappearance of jobs in industry, coupled with racial discrimination and now suspicion from the settled community regarding some religious faiths, has kept young people in lower-income urban segments, preventing them from taking advantage of emerging economic opportunities in the post-industrial economy.

Portes draws two lessons from his investigations. First, efforts to accelerate acculturation by breaking up immigrant communities and pressuring young people to give up their language to learn English can backfire since such moves drive a wedge between parents and children, reduces parental authority and promotes what might be called 'dissonant acculturation'. In this situation children and young people are deprived of the single social resource they have in tackling major discriminatory barriers.

Second, the de facto policy of admitting large numbers of poor immigrants to fill the labour needs of the economy and then subjecting them to widespread persecution is deeply flawed. It means children being raised within very low-income families with parents engaged in menial, low-paid work. Portes suggests 'selective acculturation' achieved through local groups bringing together schools, immigrant families and immigrant communities: learning English but also retaining their native language; learning the host country's values but also respecting other cultures, particularly their parents'. Intensive local collaboration among a range of children's agencies and education is necessary to avoid the dangers of downward assimilation (Portes 2003). The nature of 'culture' should not be misunderstood, however. Portes argues that within such communities, culture can be regarded as 'conflicted, open, hybridizing and fluid', embodied in ritual and social exchange (Portes 2003: 43). This process confers agency and empowers different social actors in different ways: religious and secular, men, women and young people.

CASE STUDY 8.2:
MADRASSAS IN BLACKBURN

Muslim children attend religious education and study the Koran in locally run, self-funded religious schools often attached to mosques or conducted in people's homes. Blackburn Council has appointed a link worker to work with the 30 madrassas in its area, particularly around child protection issues, and to help the madrassas to define for themselves what constitutes child abuse and to carry out police checks on teachers. The work is careful and patient: it takes time to build up relationships and to help teachers see child protection issues more clearly. The madrassas are often small, totally voluntary, and rely solely on voluntary contributions; they differ enormously in ethos and in how they are run. While the madrassas were suspicious of outsider intervention, the link worker is Muslim and has himself taught in a madrassa. This proved an essential prerequisite for building trust.

OVERCOMING DIVISION AND CONFLICT

There is immense difficulty in changing minds and in maintaining open minds. We all filter out information that does not accord with our views, and this is particularly true in politics and religion. Individuals engage in discussion with others about an issue on which they agree, and tend to confirm and strengthen their views as a result. This happens in part because the individual wishes to keep their relationship and preserve their identity and self image within the group, especially where group members share a strong identity. The consequence is a 'limited argument pool' where information is curtailed. This applies particularly to the experiences of those outside the group where the trials, experiences and suffering of outsiders are ignored, minimised or otherwise discounted (Jetten and Spears 2003).

The experience in Northern Ireland highlighted the difference between 'single-identity' and 'cross-identity' approaches to community relations, each of which is appropriate in different contexts. The former helps individuals develop deeper under-standing of culture and identity and self-awareness of a paticular group before engaging in dialogue and exchanges with members of other groups. It is a useful approach particularly when there exists a wider atmosphere of antagonism, or when there are risks to cross-community approaches or when the sense of identity may be relatively weak within particular groups (Kelly and Philpott 2003).

On the other hand, work based on 'single-identity' approaches may only encourage stereotyped views of one's own culture – 'better informed bigots' – and therefore, using that approach, the aim should be to encourage greater critical self-awareness and to enable individuals to understand what is positive and what is problematic in their beliefs and values. It should build in steps to enable members of a group to recognise how and why identities are formed, to understand the notion of multiple identities and to recognise both similarities and differences with others (Kelly and Philpott 2003: 37).

BOX 8.5: EXPERIENCES IN NORTHERN IRELAND

A team from Bradford interested in pursuing community cohesion found in a visit to Northern Ireland that local research had shown how young people who have grown up in a segregated

continued

environment that engages in heavy conflict with other segments of the community are more hostile to 'others' than older generations who have engaged outside their particular community for longer.

- Compounding this is the fact that young people feel alienated from authority and from community-wide social norms, with few or no opportunities for exerting influence. This, as Jarman (2005) concludes, partly explains the specific and significant role that young people can play in generating or sustaining conflict.
- Clearly any reconciliation strategy has to focus on engaging young people and find ways to bring their voice into local decision making, for example through a youth parliament, young persons' parish council or citizenship schooling.
- Local policy-making process should be sensitive to its impact on community tensions and conflicts.
- There is local creativity in the midst of conflict amongst community organisations, among grass roots peace builders and the voluntary sector in particular.
- There are immense difficulties in promoting cross-community discussions where most people felt more confident in engaging in discussion about an issue with others who agree. As a result change is slow with no immediate results.

(Jarman 2005)

The experiences in Northern Ireland hold many lessons for a practice seeking to overcome divisions within and between communities:

- community dialogue is not promoted by remaining silent on contentious issues
- polling is a valuable tool – finding out what people are thinking and doing as well as making contact with them
- people's history projects can act as tools for critical self-reflection within and between communities
- peace and reconciliation do work to reduce fear and tension at personal and community level
- education and training need to be provided for all involved in community outreach.

There is a debate as to whether these approaches can best be obtained in work with mixed communities or with single identity communities (Pearce 2003).

Crucially, the Northern Ireland experience showed that building local knowledge is essential. Although there is a need for a broad overview of the issue of sectarian violence, there is also a need for locally specific knowledge of the problem. Surveys developed by and for local agencies, such as the District Policing Partnerships or the Community Safety Partnerships, provided vital information for the development of local strategies. The information provided by local authorities indicated a very uneven engagement with the issue of sectarian violence. The data from local surveys could be used to inform and develop more effective and joined-up strategies to address this issue. All local authorities should be encouraged to develop strategic plans in response to sectarian violence as part of their good relations duties (Jarman 2005).

As for work with perpetrators of hate crime, a range of restorative justice programmes has been developed over recent years for dealing with people sentenced for hate crime offences and for people who have been identified as perpetrators, but not convicted as such.

BOX 8.6: THE DIFFERENCE BETWEEN ANGER AND HATRED

Conflict is always part of community and neighbourhood life as groups, organisations and institutions of all kinds strive to actualise their values and interests. Dealing with conflict is an important part of community practice, particularly when working to conciliate conflicting interests and emotions. In this it is important to recognise the difference between hatred and anger – and learn to work with and harness the latter. Hatred is far more difficult to work with. It presupposes no relationship between those who hate and those who are hated. Conversely, anger between individuals or peoples does presuppose a relationship between the parties.

As Casey writes in *Pagan Virtue*:

To be angry with someone is to be disposed to rebuke him, to remonstrate with him, demand that he apologize, have him punished. One could not satisfy one's anger simply by causing another person to be harmed. One cares about his attitudes as well as acts. If one's anger cannot be appeased by apology or restitution, and if it concentrates not upon someone's attitudes and intentions, but purely on what he has done, or even on what he is, then it has ceased to be anger and has become hatred. . . . So the natural accompaniment of anger, as well as the desire to rebuke and punish, is forgiveness. The angry man claims that his feelings and attitudes be taken seriously. He makes certain claims, and considers himself justified. Anger and apology are concerned with claims, justification, recompense.

(Casey 1991: 12–13)

Casey's all-important conclusion is that anger, though it seeks punishment and retribution, does so 'under the aspect of "the good" and of justice. Hatred on the other hand seeks to harm its object "under the aspect of evil".' In the thrall of hatred, Casey argues, a person may simply wish that 'the person one hates cease to exist' (Casey 1991: 13). He writes:

Hatred can be a lingering state existing in a subterraneous form, breaking out occasionally while anger makes certain demands and seeks a certain response. One who hates can be expected to harm the person he hates if he has the opportunity. Yet it is curiously passive. It is possible to hate without confronting directly the object of that hatred. Hatred is static, not dynamic: no claim need be made against the person who is hated and there is no expectation of a claim being recognised by that person. An apology is not relevant to hatred: if an apology does not lessen or diminish one's anger, it is not anger but hatred.

(Casey 1991: 21)

continued

Thus anger can be channelled and used, and if so it becomes productive. Loss of this perspective, however, in relation to those completely remote from us or who have vastly more power, simply produces rage – often impotent, senseless, reckless speech and void of relationship.

Anger entails reacting to someone personally, setting a value on his attitudes and intentions. It implies treating him as an agent capable of accepting or rejecting reasons for action. And that means treating him as free.

(Casey 1991: 15)

To learn to articulate my anger – and hence to feel it as anger rather than as dumb resentment – may be to introduce an active quality into what I would otherwise simply suffer. In entertaining the active emotion of anger towards someone I imply that we are both part of the same moral universe, that an exchange between us is possible, that rage may be assuaged by apology and restitution.

(Casey 1991: 21)

MEDIATION AND CONFLICT RESOLUTION

At a community level (as at an international level) mediation aims to resolve profound differences between groups in which antagonism seems to form around the very elements of life that protagonists hold most dear – their feeling of safety in their own home, the freedom to uphold cultural and religious values they prize particularly in raising their children, and their norms for creating a good and just society. As a set of techniques and approaches it has been widely embraced by central and local government as those authorities attempt to broker solutions to some of Britain's most powerful urban conflicts. It is clear that these skills are not simply to be held by one or two experts in a locality but should be spread and ready across a range of services and practitioners (NRU 2005).

First steps in mediation

1.   Decide when and how to enter the dispute. Recognise that what the mediator does at the beginning and how she or he does it will affect future activity. The mediator finds an appropriate access point and gains acceptance by parties to the conflict.
2.   Define the role. This role is not defined by law or practice; the mediator must work with those in conflict to determine exactly what that role will be. To assume that parties know what the mediator does invites misunderstanding, mistrust and failure.
3.   To make a difference the mediator must find ways to exert influence with the parties in order to meet objectives that the mediator has set. The role is not confined to simply relaying messages but must use forms of relational power.

Listening for interests

Conflicts occur when people believe that something important to them is threatened. These important, vital concerns are what mediators call 'interests'. The term can embrace both fundamental values or things which to those outside a highly personal dispute can appear trivial. In terms of communal divides it is the end of the spectrum which concerns us: deep values associated with family, children, customs and religion. Attentive listening is stock in trade for any social worker; *exactly* those same elements apply to mediating community disputes.

Understanding interests is not straightforward and often people in conflict themselves need to follow a path to explore what their core interests actually are. But there are cues provided by parties in a process of community dialogue:

- what matters to people: practically, emotionally and socially
- what they most hope to resolve
- the effect the problem has on their daily life and on their spirit
- what specific issues cause anger, upset, sense of threat and hostility
- countervailing emotions that are positive, caring and generous that have the potential to move beyond the welter of conflict and accusation (Beer and Stief 1997).

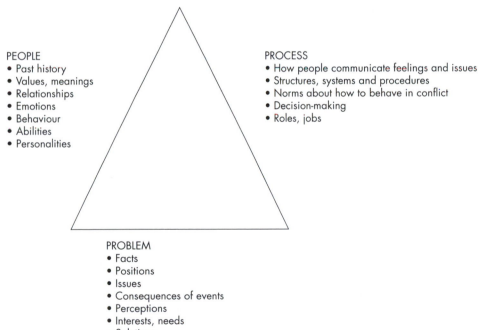

PEOPLE
- Past history
- Values, meanings
- Relationships
- Emotions
- Behaviour
- Abilities
- Personalities

PROCESS
- How people communicate feelings and issues
- Structures, systems and procedures
- Norms about how to behave in conflict
- Decision-making
- Roles, jobs

PROBLEM
- Facts
- Positions
- Issues
- Consequences of events
- Perceptions
- Interests, needs
- Solutions
- Consequences of possible outcomes

FIGURE 8.1 The conflict triangle
Adapted from Beer and Stief 1997

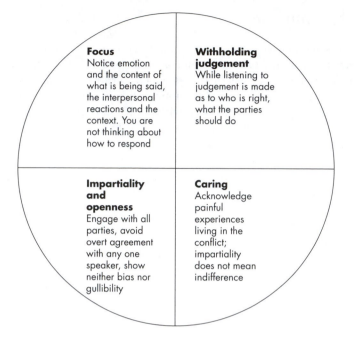

FIGURE 8.2 Attentive listening
Adapted from Beer and Stief 1997

Learning to assess which interests matter most and which can be realistically discussed is crucial to successful conflict resolution. Working on solutions means people see those interests more broadly and can separate them from a fixed position they may have adapted.

BOX 8.7: SCENARIO BUILDING

Scenario building has proven to be an important tool in the mediation process. It helps participants in a workshop clarify the consequences of their position by putting the question 'If you were to get what you wish for, what would be the consequences for you, local people and your community?'

An example comes from a workshop on the police in Northern Ireland. One group wanted to strengthen the powers and armaments of the Royal Ulster Constabulary by lifting the legal restraints and give them full backing to lock up drug dealers. Exploring the consequences of this position exposed some of the difficulties with it – the dangers of a non-accountable police force, the need for legal process and the likely community responses, among others – but it was up to the participants to decide whether or not they wanted to maintain their position.

Part of the scenario building in effect asked: 'If you get what you really want, will you then be happy, or will you want something better?' or 'How will getting what you want impact on your day-to-day life?' This raised practical issues about health care, for example, either in the context of Northern Ireland remaining in the UK or joining a united Ireland.

The scenario building was only possible after initial positions had been laid out and defended, and after people began to talk at a deeper level about their experiences, values, emotions, fears and hopes. Working on scenarios earlier in the process would have led to more people simply defending their positions.

A further stage of the scenario building was to ask if there were alternative goals that appealed to people (it was up to participants, not facilitators, to suggest answers), or alternative ways to achieve these goals. This also opened up discussion of the likely consequences of the goals of other groups and whether alternatives were possible for them or not.

BOX 8.8: THE QUAKERS' LONG AND SUCCESSFUL RECORD IN MEDIATING DISPUTES

The Quakers have had one of the longest and most respected track records in mediating the toughest, most entrenched conflicts over values, home and family. They have three conditions for entering into mediation efforts: i) total anonymity for the intervention, ii) each party having a veto over continuing the process at any point, and iii) no deadline. These conditions say two things. One, that:

> this is your dispute, not ours. The communication and reconciliation that may happen is also yours and not ours. You will have complete control over the process in the sense that you can single-handedly cancel it at any time.
>
> (Kolb *et al.* 1994: 454)

Second that we, as mediators have no reputation to enhance and no interest in the outcome other than that we would like to see violence end and peace achieved. Moreover, we are here for the duration of the process and will focus on specific proposals only when the parties are ready and suggest them themselves.

These conditions render Quaker mediators 'powerless' in one sense: they have no blandishments, rewards or threats of pain to deploy. But it also renders them powerful in the sense that it sets the standards for intervention and how the parties must react one to another if the mediation process is to go forward: parties can refrain from accusing each other of bad faith because they need not fear looking weak; they can reveal deeper worries or ponder alternative solutions with low risk of losing face. Above all it can provide an outlet for conciliatory and non-belligerent gestures.

> (Kolb *et al.* 1994: 456)

Community dialogue

The organisation Community Dialogue believes that the experiences and feelings underpinning the positions which people hold are at least as important as the substantive positions themselves, and aims to overcome conflict at that level. This framework allows people to move beyond immobilising issues such as whether the only effective work is across all sections of a community divide. The organisation does not find terms like 'cross-community', 'single identity' or 'community relations' helpful or particularly relevant in its work. Some of the dialogues it organises are for specific communities, groups or individuals. Some of the dialogues are for diverse communities, groups or individuals. In general terms some of the dialogues are reflective of particular interest groups (for example human rights) or specific identifies (for example Loyalists) and some are representative of more diverse interest groups and identities (Lennon 2004).

But neither does the organisation avoid the issues at the heart of conflict. Doing so allows parties to pretend that there is no conflict, suggesting to others that the mediator does not care. To ignore issues allows the conflict either to simmer and grow or reinforces the notion that conflict is terrible and best avoided, when in fact it can be a necessary catalyst for a solution.

BOX 8.9:   COMMUNITY DIALOGUE: TOOLS AND TECHNIQUES

Dialogue:

- Is a process involving active listening as well as talking. It also implies accepting and respecting the views of others and trying to understand where they are coming from. Diversity and division are openly addressed in this process.
- Deepens understanding of the parties' positions, often leading to shared understanding and an enhancement of the ability to make informed decisions.
- Shifts the focus from the stated positions that parties so often argue over to the needs (often shared), which underlie them. It achieves this by getting people to question their own positions and those of others and to look at the needs underlying them.

In this process straightforward questions are asked of the parties: What is it you want? What do you really need and why do you need it? What could you live with, given that the needs and hopes of others may differ from yours?

The process has clear ground rules:

Trust – take the chance to share feelings and experiences with other people though this may make some people feel uncomfortable. The past experience of the process indicates that this is a calculated risk that is worth taking.

Confidentiality – participants often share sensitive information and this may lead to difficulties for those participants and damage the credibility of the process if total confidence is not respected. This means that no attributable comments should be shared with anyone outside of the boundaries in which they were heard, and this includes not telling others the names of people who were present.

Acceptance – of the right of an individual to hold beliefs you regard as wrong is different from respecting those beliefs. All participant's contributions and ideas have value.

Respect – dialogue can involve dealing with people whose beliefs some may feel cannot be respected because they are utterly wrong. Persons taking part do not have to respect the beliefs that they consider wrong but should treat all participants with the same level of respect that they themselves would want. This means that parties should separate the beliefs (and actions flowing from those beliefs) from the person who holds them. Persons taking part do not have to hide a dislike of what they hear, however, because dialogue has no value without honesty.

(adapted from Holloway 2004)

KEY POINTS

☐   There has been appreciable concern within urban centres and government that there are growing communal divides, if not outright segregation based on faith and ethnicity.

☐   Religious belief is sometimes seen as a prominent source of communal division but also offers many resources for community development and building social capital. Social work has only partially engaged in its understanding of religion and its impact on communities; the notion of 'spirituality' is a beginning but does not produce clear cut pathways for practitioners interested in spanning community divides.

☐   Government community cohesion policies put considerable responsibilities on communities to take positive steps to finding a common set of values.

☐   There is a range of processes around mediation and dialogue that community practitioners should be engaging in if they are to play their part in overcoming division and strife when it is present in the communities in which they work.

CHAPTER 9

DISCUSSION ON THE ACTIVITIES

ACTIVITY 1.1: IDENTIFYING NEIGHBOURHOOD CHARACTERISTICS (11)

Our understanding of what defines a specific neighbourhood is more subjective and personal than you might think. In other words two neighbours living side by side could have very different views as to where the neighbourhood begins and ends. This activity is simply aimed at getting you to begin to define for yourself the neighbourhood in which you work or live. Having developed your idea of the specific neighbourhood you have in mind, an interesting further step would be to consult a colleague or neighbour where you live to see if he or she agrees with your sense of 'the neighbourhood'.

ACTIVITY 1.2: HOW FAR CAN PRACTITIONERS TACKLE NEIGHBOURHOOD DISADVANTAGE? (12)

This activity probes how far your agency might *actually* be willing to commit itself to delivering community-based services in collaboration with other local agencies aimed at tackling disadvantage holistically. While service organisations, whether local authority, health based or voluntary, adopt the rhetoric of community-based services, they often commit resources only to dealing with their specific group of users. As a consequence they fail to free up the staff time and resources to develop closer contact with local people and organisations necessary to tackle the large problems in concert.

ACTIVITY 2.1: SITUATING SERVICE AGENCIES IN NEIGHBOURHOOD AND COMMUNITY (25)

The aim here is to get you thinking about the other service providers in your locality: how neighbourhood-focused are they, and how committed are they to having local people participate in shaping the development of their service? Think of the entire range of agencies at work in your locality, including faith and cultural institutions, who may have a role to play.

ACTIVITY 2.2: USING THE NATIONAL STATISTICS DATABASE (35)

What does the data tell you about the neighbourhood? Think in terms of the kinds of social problems the data may be indicating are present. Does the data allow you to infer what the dominant problems for residents might be?

ACTIVITY 3.1: WHAT IS THE BALANCE OF POWER WITHIN THE COLLABORATIVE? (50)

It is worth investing some time in developing a full list of local organisations for this activity. Do some quick research, that is consult a register of organisations if you have one available or simply set aside time to think broadly about all the organisations that might be interested in joining in a service delivery partnership. Don't forget faith-based organisations, small community groups run by volunteers such as low-cost day centres for older people, youth centres, and residents' associations among many.

ACTIVITY 3.2: SEX WORKERS IN THE LOCALITY: HOW TO RESPOND? (53)

This case study is a good example of the kind of contemporary social problem that services and practitioners are having to grapple with and one, moreover, with no easy answers. It is the kind of problem that has conflicting moral dimensions and extends across professional remits. How it is resolved has consequences for the women (and for any children that may be involved), and has child protection implications if the women are under 18. It also has implications for community safety and how local people live their lives. Any response is going to be less than perfect. Yet some response is necessary since the situation cannot be allowed to drift.

As revealed in the research referred to in the case study, the sex workers' greatest concern was for a safe working environment. Improving relations with street workers then is a high priority, as is helping them cope with their immediate situation through mediation and awareness-raising. Another step would be to involve sex workers in local governance of any proposed responses, which would help ensure consideration of their needs when addressing community conflicts and managing the street scene. But neither can the community's concerns be ignored. The survey indicated that 'Co-existence was greatest where integrated responses to community concerns had been developed with a range of partners including sex support projects and where alternatives to increased enforcement such as court diversion schemes existed.'

ACTIVITY 3.3: PARTNERSHIP IN ACTION (60)

This activity probes the difficulty of maintaining partnerships when organisations are seriously trying to deliver a neighbourhood-level service with a local face. Such a way of working challenges senior managers' sense of control. Conflicting levels of political authority may well exacerbate partnership working: for example a shire county agency may have trouble linking through to its personnel involved in a neighbourhood management programme overseen by a city council. (This was actually the case with the constabulary in this example.) There are no easy solutions to resolving such emphatic disagreement. You may have to draft in a senior officer from your own agency – if you can. Conversely, if the police in this case had entered into a partnership understanding and there were agreed targets or public service agreements, perhaps revisiting those with discussions might have resolved the issue.

ACTIVITY 4.1: STRATEGY CHART (69)

The concept of community development may cause you some uncertainty since it draws on radical political theorising from the 1970s like Paulo Freire and aims to give local people more 'voice' and more influence in local affairs – in a word, more power. This activity asks you to think pragmatically and in a hard-headed way about how to obtain certain objectives for your organisation when it is joining in campaigns to change local thinking or win greater concessions in terms of the rights of local service users. Disability organisations and women concerned with domestic abuse have used such campaigning methods to great effect – an example of what can be achieved.

ACTIVITY 4.2: PUBLIC MEETINGS: SOME DRAWBACKS (74) AND ACTIVITY 4.3 HOW TO GUARANTEE A POOR MEETING (76)

Practitioners spend a great deal of time in meetings and they are also often responsible for arranging meetings with community groups or with the public at large. Yet meetings frequently achieve very little and fritter away a lot of time. Who has not groaned inwardly when sitting in a PowerPoint presentation it is clear that there are still another twenty slides to go or when a speaker who has already had the floor three times rises to make another point – irrelevant to all but him or her?

These activities are designed to get you to reflect on how meetings might be better run – both meetings with other colleagues and professionals and with the public. They do this by getting you to focus on all the things that can go wrong and derail a meeting. By combining these ideas with the text in this section hopefully you can construct and take part in more productive meetings.

ACTIVITY 5.1: THE DIFFICULTIES IN FOCUSING ON OUTCOMES (90)

Progress towards outcomes, and not just lip-service, is absolutely critical to delivering locally oriented services that people want and increasingly expect. All initiatives or pieces of work should be looked at in terms of how they may have progressed in relation to the five outcomes from *Every Child Matters*. Outcomes are what we want for all our children, and there is still much thinking to do in relation to how the concept of outcomes will change the work we do. They are emphatically *not* another target or performance measurement.

ACTIVITY 6.1: WHAT IS ANTI-SOCIAL BEHAVIOUR? (114)

The figures in the survey were as follows: Rowdy teenagers on the streets/youths hanging around: 71 per cent; drug dealing: 63 per cent; noisy neighbours: 44 per cent; mugging: 44 per cent; burglary: 42 per cent; graffiti: 34 per cent; speeding: 34 per cent; traffic noise and pollution: 22 per cent.

ACTIVITY 6.2: COLLABORATING IN LOCAL ACTION ON ANTI-SOCIAL BEHAVIOUR (116)

This activity simply encourages practitioners to either develop or find out what exactly constitutes anti-social behaviour as far as the agency they work for is concerned. It means different things to different people – but working with other agencies in tackling anti-social behaviour will be difficult unless all concerned can agree on what are the priority behaviours that need to be tackled. Do not make the list too long. In the Blacon area of Chester burnt-out cars were viewed by residents as the number one manifestation of anti-social behaviour, and the Neighbourhood Management Pathfinder in that area, which had close links to the community, made it their number one priority and successfully curtailed the number of cars that were set on fire.

It is interesting that burglary featured so low in comparison to youths hanging around in groups. But this has been confirmed more than once – the public views young people in groups as incredibly threatening.

ACTIVITY 6.3: HOW LIKELY WOULD NEIGHBOURS BE TO INTERVENE IF . . .? (117)

This activity probes the willingness of local people to get involved, in other words to maintain a sense of informal social control and to uphold certain informal norms of behaviour. Many researchers and policymakers, not to mention government itself, see this as a key element in maintaining what we used to call 'community spirit'. Without it, the argument goes, the sense of authority is lost and anti-social behaviour even in younger children is able to flourish. You may agree or disagree with this proposition – it is certainly worth debating.

As for the results of the Family and Neighbourhood Survey (FANS) on the willingness of local people to get involved the results were logged on a scale of 1–5, with 1 indicating the lowest willingness to get involved and 5 the highest: 4.3 has a knife; 4.2 taking something from house, garage or garden; 4.1 playing with matches; 4.1 spray paints or writes on a building or car; 4.0 left alone in the evening; 4.0 throws rocks at another child; 3.9 left alone during the day; 3.9 shoplifting; 3.8 falls off bike; 3.6 throws rocks at a dog; 3.4 wandering by himself/herself; 3.1 hits a child the same age; 2.6 being spanked by an adult in the street; 2.5 picks flowers from a garden. When I do this exercise with students their opinions of their own neighbours' willingness to get involved is generally far lower on the scale.

ACTIVITY 6.4: EDUCATIONAL ATTAINMENT OF LOOKED-AFTER YOUNG PEOPLE (128)

This is a key statistic opening a window on what happens to young people in care in your area. In general it is important to keep public service targets in mind and to check on progress (or lack of it) towards achieving them.

ACTIVITY 6.5: HOMELESSNESS AND YOUNG OFFENDERS (129)

This activity encourages you to reflect on a fast-growing problem that will affect some localities quite sharply.

ACTIVITY 7.1: IDENTIFYING NETWORKS (141)

This activity is self-explanatory – but that does not make it easy. As this chapter explains, networks of older people can thin out dramatically for a host of reasons. However, practitioners must not assume this nor cease in efforts to bolster or augment what networks an older person may have that they are working with.

ACTIVITY 7.2: IS CHOICE EASY? (142)

'Choice' has become something of a mantra both from government and service agencies themselves. Sometimes the word is used simply as a cover for other changes, which may in fact include a reduction of actual service. The objective of this activity is to get you to think about how difficult making choices about different service options can be for any individual and for older people in particular. The activity aims to get you to empathise fully with the person who has to make the decision. It is not easy in a service environment of multiple social care providers, fragmented lines of communication among agencies and the continuous constriction of resources.

ACTIVITY 7.3: SOCIAL CARE ASSESSMENT AND DECISION MAKING (143)

This activity, linked to the one above, underscores the considerable cost pressures that constrain and will continue to constrain a once-comprehensive local public provision.

ACTIVITY 8.1: A TEST FOR CITIZENSHIP? (155)

This activity asks a searching question: are there certain fundamentals of citizenship that all citizens can agree on and should uphold? Should these fundamental commitments then be expected of all who aim to become citizens in the UK? If so, what might these be? Should the command of the English language be one of them? Knowing the constitution of the United Kingdom? In a period when recent surveys have reported a *decline* in 'Britishness' (as devolution encourages an identity based on the individual nations making up the United Kingdom) where does this leave the idea of common ideals?

REFERENCES

Acheson, D. (1998) *Independent Inquiry into Inequalities in Health*, London, TSO

Adams, R. (2003) *Social Work and Empowerment*, Third Edition, Basingstoke, Palgrave Macmillan

Ahmed, R. (2000) *The Role of Faith Based Organisations in Community Development*, CCWA briefing 27, Churches' community Work Alliance, Durham

Ai, A. (2002) Integrating spirituality into professional education: a challenging but feasible task, *Journal of Teaching in Social Work* 22, 1/2: 103–130

Aldgate, J., Jones, D., Rose, W. and Jeffery, C. (2006) *The Developing World of the Child*, London, Jessica Kingsley Publishers

Allen, J. (2004) The Whereabouts of Power: Politics, Government and Space *Geografiska Annaler, Series B: Human Geography* 86, 1: 19–32

—— (2003) *Lost Geographies of Power*, Oxford, Blackwell

Audit Commission (2004) *Older People – independence and well-being: the Challenge for public services*, London, Audit Commission

Axford, N. and Berry, V. (2005) Measuring Outcomes in the 'New' Childrens' Services, *Journal of Integrated Care* 13: 12–23

Bailey, R. and Brake M. [eds] (1975) *Radical Social Work*, London, Edward Arnold

Banja, J. (1995) *Religiosity and spirituality among persons with disabilities: Application to rehabilitation environments*, A draft paper for the Fetzer Foundation, Michigan, Kalamazoo

Banks, S., Butcher, H., Henderson, P. and Robertson, J. (2003) *Managing Community Practice: Principles, Policies and Programmes*, Bristol, Policy Press

Barber, B. (2003) *Strong Democracy: Participatory Politics for New Age*, London, University of California Press

Barclay, P. (1982) *Social Work: Roles, Tasks and Responsibilities*, London, Bedford Press

Bardach, E. (2005) *A Practical Guide for Policy Analysis: The Eightfold Path to More Effective Problem Solving*, Washington DC, Congressional Quarterly Press

Barnes, J. (2006a) *What prevents, or could increase, informal social control in neighbourhoods?* London, London School of Economics/CASE seminar

Barnes, J., Katz, I., Korbin, J. and O'Brien, M. (2006) *Children and Families in Communities: Theory, Research, policy and practice*, Chichester, John Wiley and Sons

Bauder, H. (2001) Work, Young People and Neighbourhood Representations. *Social and Cultural Geography* 2: 46–480

Bauman, Z. (2001) *Community -Seeking Safety in an Insecure World*, Cambridge, Polity Press

Beck, U. (1992) *The Risk Society*, London, Sage

Beer, J. and Stief, E. (1997) *The Mediator's Handbook*, Gabriola Island, BC, New Society Publishers

Bellefeuille, D. and Hemingway, D. (2005) The new politics of community-based governance requires a fundamental shift in the nature and character of the administrative bureaucracy. *Children and Youth Services Review* 27: 491–498

Benn, M. (2005) No Status with Age, *Community Care*, 16–22 June

Bentley, T. and Gurumurthy, R. (1999) *Destination Unknown: Engaging with the problems of marginalised youth*, London, Demos

Blacon Neighbourhood Management Pathfinder (2005) *Community Engagement Checklist*, Chester, Icarus Collective Ltd

Blears, H. (2004) *The Politics of Decency*, London, Mutuo

Bobo, K., Kendal, J. and Max, S. (2000) *Organizing for Social Change*: Midwest Academy Manual for Activists, Minneapolis, Seven Locks Press

Boylan, P. (2006) *The Virtual Child: A Presentation* Chester, Blacon Neighbourhood Management Pathfinder

Boylan, P., Pierson, J. and Thomas, M. (2006) *Blacon is Working: Achievements and Prospects of the Neighbourhood Management Pathfinder*, Chester, Blacon Neighbourhood Management Pathfinder

Boutall, T. and Pollet, S. (2003) A Standards Framework for Managing Volunteers. *Journal of Volunteer Administration* 21: 5–12

Bowles, S. and Gintis, H. (2002) Social Capital and Community Governance. *The Economic Journal* 112: F419–436

Boxall, M. (2002) *Nurture Groups in School: Principles and Practice*, London, Paul Chapman Publishing

Bracht, N. (1999) *Health Promotion at the Community Level*, London, Sage Publications

Braithwaite, J. (2001) Restorative Justice and a New Criminal Law of Substance Abuse. *Youth and Society* 33: 227–248

Bremner, J. (2005) Will Prevention Be a Cure-All? *Community Care*, 9–15 June

Briggs, X. (1997) Social Capital and the Cities: Advice to Change Agents, Bellagio, Italy, International Workshop on Community Building

—— (2002) *The Will and the Way: Local Partnerships, Political Strategy and the Well Being of American's Children and Youth*, Cambridge, Mass, Harvard University Faculty Resource Working Papers

—— (2004) *Traps and Stepping Stones: Neighbourhood Dynamics and Family Well-being* Cambridge, Mass, Harvard University Faculty Resource Working Papers

British Association of Social Workers (2006) *Response to DfES Consultation on Budget Holding Lead Professionals*, Birmingham, BASW

Brody, G., Murray, V., Ge, X., Kim, S., Simons, R., Gibbons, F., Gerrard, M. and Conger, D. (2003) Neighborhood Disadvantage Moderates Associations of Parenting and Older Sibling Problem Attitudes and Behaviour With Conduct Disorders in African American Children. *Journal of Consulting and Clinical Psychology* 71: 211–222

Brooks-Gunn, J., Duncan, G., Aber, L. eds. (1997) *Neighborhood Poverty: Context and Consequences for Children*, New York, Russell Sage Foundation

Bronfenbrenner, U. (1979) *The Ecology of Human Development*, Cambridge, Mass, Harvard University Press

Browning, C., Cagney, K. (2002) Neighborhood Structural Disadvantage, Collective Efficacy, and Self-Rated Physical Health in an Urban Setting. *Journal of Health and Social Behavior* 43: 388–399

Bunting, M. (2006) It takes more than tea and biscuits to overcome indifference and fear, *The Guardian*, November 13

—— (2006a) In our angst over children we're ignoring the perils of adulthood, *The Guardian*, February 27

Burns, D., Heywood, F., Taylor, M., Wilde, P. and Wilson, M. (2004) *Making community participation meaningful*, Bristol, Policy Press

Cabinet Office (2000) *National Strategy for Neighbourhood Renewal: a Framework for Consultation*, London, HMSO

Cannan, C. and Warren, C. (1997) *Social Action with Children and Families: A Community Development Approach to Child and Family Welfare*, London, Routledge

Carneiro, P. and Heckman, J. (2003) Human Capital Policy, in Heckman, J. and Krueger, A. [ed.], *Inequality in America: What role for Human Capital Policities?* Cambridge Mass, The MIT Press

Carrier, J. (2005) *Older People, the New Agenda* Presentation to Better Government for Older People Network, London

Casey, J. (1991) *Pagan Virtue An Essay in Ethics*. Oxford, Clarendon

Central council for education and training in social work (1991) *Rules and Requirements for the Diploma in Social Work* Paper 30, London, CCETSW

Challis, D., Darton, R., Johnson, L. and Stone, M. (1988) Services, Resource Management and the Integration of Health and Social Care in Cambridge, in P. Knapp, M. (eds) *Demonstrating Successful Care in the Community*, Canterbury, PSSRU

Chambers, E. (2004) *Roots for Radicals Organizing for Power, Action and Justice*, New York and London, Continuum International Publishing

Chaskin, R., Brown, P., Venkatesh, S. and Vidal, A. (2001) *Building Community Capacity*, New York, Aldine de Gruyter, Hawthorne

Ciulla, J. (2004) *The Ethics of Leadership*, New York, Praeger

Clark, K. and Drinkwater, S. (2002) Enclaves, Neighbourhood Effects and Employment Outcomes: Ethnic Minorities in England and Wales, *Journal of Population Economics* 15: 5–29

Clayden, J. and Stein, M. (2005) *Mentoring Young People Leaving Care: 'Someone for me'*, York, Joseph Rowntree Foundation

Cohen, D., Bedimo, A., Scribner, R., Basolo, V. and Farley, T. (2003) Neighborhood Physical Conditions and Health, *American Journal of Public Health* 93: 467–471

Collinshaw, S., Maugha, B. and Goodman, R. (2004) Time Trends in Adolescent Mental Health, *Journal of Child Psychology and Psychiatry* 45: 1350–1362

Craig, G., Taylor, M., Szanto, C. and Wilkinson, M. (1999) *Developing Local Compacts: Relationships Between Local Public Sector Bodies and the Voluntary and Community Sectors*, York, York Publishing Service

Craig, G., Taylor, M., Wilkinson, M. and Bloor, K. with Munro, S. and Syed, A. (2002) *Contract or Trust? The Role of Compacts in Local Governance*, Bristol, The Policy Press

Craig, G., Taylor, M., Carlton, N., Garbutt, R., Kimberlee, R., Lepine, E. and Syed, A. (2005) *The Paradox of Compacts: Monitoring the Impact of Compacts*, London, Home Office

Crimmens, D., Factor, F., Jeffs, T., Pitts, J., Pugh, C., Spence, J. and Turner, P. (2004) *Reaching Socially Excluded Young People: A National Study of Street-based Youth Work*, Leicester, National Youth Agency

Crist, J. (2005) The Meaning for Elders of Receiving Family Care, *Journal of Advanced Nursing*, 49, 5: 485–493

Cummings, T. (1984) Trans-organizational Development, *Research in Organizational Behavior* 6: 367–422

Cunningham, B. (1998) Recruiting Male Volunteers to Build Staff Diversity: Men in Child Care, *Child Care Information Exchange*: 20–22

Dalrymple, J. and Burke, B. (1995) *Anti-Oppressive Practice: Social Care and the Law*, Buckingham, Open University Press

Daniel, B., Featherstone, B., Hooper, C. and Scourfield, J. (2005) Why Gender Matters for Every Child Matters, *British Journal of Social Work* 35, 8: 1343–1355

Daniel, B. and Wassell, S. (2002) *Adolescence: Assessing and Promoting Resilience in Vulnerable Children*, London, Jessica Kingsley Publishers

Davey, B., Levin, E., Iliffe, S. and Kharicha, K. (2005) Integrating Health and Social Care: Implications for Joint Working and Community Care Outcomes for Older People, *Journal of Interprofessional Care* 19, 1: 22–34

Delgado, M. (2000) *Community Social Work Practice in an Urban Context*, New York, Oxford University Press

Department for Education and Skills (2002) *National Drugs Strategy: Tackling Drugs to Build a Better Britain*, DfES

—— (2003) *The Impact of Parental Involvement, Parental Support and Family Education on Pupil Achievement and Adjustment: A Literature Review*, London, DfES

—— (2004) *Common Assessment Framework: Consultation*, London, DfES

—— (2005a) *Higher Standards, Better Schools for All – More Choice for Parents and Pupils*, London, DfES

—— (2005b) *Youth Matters*, London, DfES

—— (2006) *Statistics of Education: Outcome Indicators for Looked After Children – 12 months to 30 September 2005*, London, DfES

Department of Health (1998) *Our Healthier Nation*, London, DoH

—— (2000a) *The NHS Plan*, London, The Stationery Office

—— (2000b) *Framework for the Assessment of Children in Need and their Families*, London, TSO

—— (2001a) *Intermediate Care*, London, DoH

—— (2001b) *National Service Framework for Older People*, London, DoH

—— (2004) *Recognising and Managing Depression in Residents of Aged Care Homes*, London, DoH

—— (2005a) *Supporting People with Long Term Conditions: An NHS and Social Care Model to Support Local Innovation and Integration*, London, DoH

—— (2005b) *National Standards, Local Action: Health and Social Care Standards and Planning Framework 2005–8*, London, DoH

—— (2005c) *Independence, Well-being and Choice: Our Vision for the Future of Social Care for Adults*, London, TSO

—— (2006a) *Our Health, Our Care, Our Say*, London, DoH

—— (2006b) *A New Ambition for Old Age: Next Steps in Implementing the National Service Framework for Older People*, London, DoH

Dettmer, P., Thurston, L. and Dyck, N. (2001) *Consultation, Collaboration and Teamwork for Students with Special Needs*, New York, Allyn and Bacon

Dietz, R. (2002) The Estimation of Neighborhood Effects in the Social Sciences: An Interdisciplinary Approach, *Social Science Research* 31: 539–575

Diez-Roux, A. (2001) Investigating Neighborhood and Area Effects on Health, *American Journal of Public Health* 91: 1783–1789

Dowling, B., Powell, M. and Glendinning, C. (2004) Conceptualising Successful Partnerships. *Health and Social Care in the Community* 12, 4: 309–317

Dubois, W.E.B. (1903) *The Souls of Black Folk*, Chicago, A.C.McClurg & Co

Easen, P., Atkins, M. and Dyson, A. (2000) Professional Collaboration and Conceptualisation of Practice, *Children and Society* 14: 355–367

Edwards, M. and Gaventa, J. (eds) (2000) *Global Citizen Action*, London, Earthscan

Ewing, R., Govekar, M., Govekar, P. and Rishi, M. (2002) Economics, Market Segmentation and Recruiting: Targeting Your Promotion to Volunteers' Needs, *Journal of Nonprofit and Public Sector Marketing* 10: 63–96

Farnell, R., Furbey, R., Shams, S., Hills, Al-Haqq, Macey, M. and Smith, G. (2003) *'Faith' in urban regeneration? Engaging faith communities in urban regeneration*, Bristol, The Policy Press

Farver, J. and Natera, L. (2000) Effects of Neighborhood Violence on Preschoolers' Social Function with Peers, *International Perspectives on Child and Adolescent Mental Health*, Volume 1: Proceedings of the First International Conference: 42–57

Feinstein, L. (2003) Inequality in the Early Cognitive Development of British Children in the 1970 Cohort, *Economica* 70: 73–97

—— (2007) *The role of education in reducing inequality*, Presentation to the conference, Commission on Families and the Well-being of Children, February 16

Flint, J. (2002) Return of the Governors: Citizenship and the New Governance of Neighbourhood Disorder in the UK, *Citizenship Studies* 6: 245–264

Flores, J., Montgomery, S. and Lee, S. (2005) Organization and Staffing Barriers to Parent Involvement in Teen Pregnancy, *Journal of Adolescent Health* 37, 3, SUPP, S108–S114

Flynn, S. (2005) A Sociocultural Perspective on an Inclusive Framework for the Assessment of Children with an Autistic Spectrum Disorder within Mainstream Settings, *Educational and Child Psychology* 22: 39–49

Folgheraiter, R. (2004) *Relational Social Work: Toward Networking and Societal Practices*, London, Jessica Kingsley Publishers

Foster, E. and Gifford, E. (2005) The Transition to Adulthood for Youth Leaving Public Systems: Challenges to Policies and Research, in Settersten, F., Furstenberg, F. and Rumbaut, R. (eds), *On the Frontier of Adulthood: Theory, Research and Public Policy*, Chicago, University of Chicago Press

Furbey, R., Dinham, A., Farnell, R., Finneron, D. and Wilkinson, G. (2006) *Faith as social capital: Connecting or dividing?* Bristol, The Policy Press

Furlong, A. and Cartmel, F. (2004) *Vulnerable Young Men in Fragile Labour Markets: Employment, Unemployment and the Search for Long-term Security*, York, Joseph Rowntree Foundation

Fussell, E. and Furstenberg, F. (2005) The Transition to Adulthood during the Twentieth Century: Race, Nativity, and Gender, in Settersten, R., Furstenberg, F. and Rumbaut, R. (eds), *On the Frontier of Adulthood Theory, Research and Public Policy*, Chicago, University of Chicago Press

Gerth, H. and Wright Mills, C. (eds) (2007) *From Max Weber: Essays in Sociology*, London, Routledge

Gesler, W. (1992) Therapeutic Landscapes: Medical Issues in Light of the New Cultural Geography, *Social Science and Medicine* 34: 735–746

Ghate, D. and Hazel, N. (2002) *Parenting in Poor Environments: Stress, Support and Coping*, London, Jessica Kingsley Publishers

Giddens, A. (1991) *Modernity and Self-identity: Self and Society in the Late Modern Age*, Cambridge, Polity Press

Gibbons, J., Gallagher, B., Bell, C. and Gordon, D. (1995). *Development After Physical Abuse in Early Childhood: A Follow-up Study of Children on Protection Registers*, London, HMSO

Gilan, A. (2005) Ghettoes in English cities 'almost equal to Chicago' *The Guardian*, September 23

Gilchrist, R. and Jeffs, T. (eds) (2001) *Settlements, Social Change and Community Action*, London, Jessica Kingsley Publishers

Gill, O., Tanner, C. and Bland, L. (2002) *Family Support: Strengths and Pressures in a 'High Risk' Neighbourhood*, Ilford, Barnardo's

Goldsmith, S. and Eggers, W. (2004) *Governing by Network: The New Shape of the Public Sector*, Washington DC, Brookings Institution

Greater Chesterton Neighbourhood Action Planning Project (2006) *Resources for Change: A Discussion Paper*, Newcastle under Lyme, GCNAP

Griffiths, R. (1988) *Community Care: Agenda for Action*, London, HMSO

Haines, K. and Case, S. (2005) Promoting Prevention: Targeting Family-Based Risk and Protective Factors for Drug Use and Youth Offending in Swansea, *British Journal of Social Work* 35: 169–187

Harker, L. (2005) Bounce-back, *Community Care*, 3–10 May

Harris, J. (2003) *The Social Work Business*, London, Routledge

Hayes, D. (2005) Degree of scepticism greets Ladyman's proposed course, *Community Care*, 47

Hendricks, C. and Rudich, G. (2000) A Community Building Perspective in Social Work Education, *Journal of Community Practice* 8: 21–36

Henery, N. (2003) The Reality of Visions: Contemporary Theories of Spirituality in Social Work, *British Journal of Social Work* 33: 1105–1113

Henwood, M. and Waddington, E. (2002) *Outcomes of Social Care for Adults (OSCA): Messages for Policy and Practice*, Leeds, Nuffield Institute for Health

Hill, O. (2003) *Letters to My Fellow Workers*, London, Civitas

HM Treasury (2004) *Choice for Parents, the Best Start for Children: a 10-year Strategy for Childcare*, HM Treasury, DTI, DWP

HM Treasury and Department for Education and Skills (2005) *Support for Parents: The Best Start for Children*, London, HMSO

HM Treasury, Department for Education and Skills, Department of Work and Pensions (2003) *Every Child Matters*, HMSO

Holloway, D. (2004) *A Practical Guide to Dialogue*, Belfast, Community Dialogue

Home Office (2001) *Community Cohesion: A Report of the Independent Review Team* (The Cantle Report), London, Home Office

—— (2005) *Improving Opportunity, Strengthening Society*, London, Home Office

Houston, S. (2002) Re-thinking a Systemic Approach to Child Welfare: A Critical Response to the Framework for the Assessment of Children in Need and their Families, *European Journal of Social Work* 5: 301–312

Hudson, B. (2002) Interprofessionality in Health and Social Care: The Achilles' Heel of Partnership? *Journal of Interprofessional Care* 16: 7–17

—— (2005) Interdisciplinary teams, *Community Care*, 21–28 April

Hudson, B. (2006) Integrated Team Workiing: Making the Interagency Connection, *Journal of Integrated Care* 14, 2: 26–36

Huntington, J. (1981) *Social Work and General Medical Practice: Collaboration or Conflict?* London, George Allen and Unwin

Improvement and Development Agency (2005) *Show Me How I Matter: Part 3*, London, Local Government Association

Innes, M. (2004) Signal crimes and signal disorder: notes on deviance as communicative action, *The British Journal of Sociology* 55, 3: 335–355

Institute for Public Policy Research (2005) *Mental Health in the Mainstream*, London, IPPR

International Association of Schools of Social Work (2001) *International Definition of Social Work*, IASSW

International Federation of Social Workers (2000) *Definition of Social Work* www.ifsw./org/en/ p38000208.html, accessed 23.3.07

Jack, G. and Gill, O. (2003) *The Missing Side of the Triangle: Assessing the Importance of Family and Environmental Factors in the Lives of Children*, Ilford, Barnardo's

Jack, G., Jack, D. (2000) Ecological Social Work: The Application of a Systems Model of Development in Context, in Stepney, P. and Ford, D. (eds) *Social Work Models, Methods and Theories: A Framework for Practice*, Lyme Regis, UK, Russell House

Jackson, S. (1998) Educational Success for Looked-after Children: The Social Worker's Responsibility, *Practice* 10, 4: 47–56

Jargowsky, P. (1996) *Poverty and Place: Ghettos, Barrios, and the American City*, New York, Russell Sage Foundation

Jarman, N. (2005) *No Longer A Problem: Sectarian Violence in Northern Ireland*, Belfast, Institute for Conflict Research

Jenkins, S. (2004) *Big Bang Localism: A Rescue Plan for British Democracy*, London, Policy Exchange

Jetten, J. and Spears, R. (2003) The Divisive Potential of Differences and Similarities: The Role of Intergroup Distinctiveness in Intergroup Differentiation, *European Review of Social Psychology* 14: 203–241

Jimoul, L. (2006) *The Art of Politics: Broad-base Organising in Britain*, PhD thesis, Queen Mary, University of London

Jones, C., Ferguson, I., Lavalette, M. and Penketh, L. (2005) *Social Work and Social Justice: A*

Manifesto for a New Engaged Practice, http://www.liv.ac.uk/ssp/Social_Work_Manifesto. html, accessed January 16 2006

Jones, G. (2002) *The Youth Divide: Diverging Paths to Adulthood*, York, York Publishing Society

Kaner S. with Lind, L., Toldi, C., Fisk, S. and Berger, D. (1996) *Facilitator's Guide to Participatory Decision-Making*, British Columbia, New Society Publishers

Keating, N., Otfinowski, P., Wenger, C., Fast, J. and Derksen, L. (2003) Understanding the Caring Capacity of Informal Networks of Frail Seniors: A Case for Care Nnetworks, *Ageing and Society* 23: 115–127

Kelling, G. and Wilson, J. (1982) Broken Windows, *Atlantic Monthly*, 29–38

Kelly, R. and Philpott, S. (2003) *Community Cohesion – Moving Bradford Forward: Lessons from Northern Ireland*, Bradford, University of Bradford and Government Office for Yorkshire and Humber

Kenyon, E. (2002) *Young Adults' Household Formation: Individualisation, Identity and Home*. Exploration in Sociology Conference Proceedings

Kharicha, K., Iliffe, S., Levin, E., Davey, B. and Fleming, C. (2005) Tearing Down the Berlin Wall: Social Workers' Perspectives on Joint Working with General Practice, *Family Practice* 22: 399–405

Kharicha, K., Levin, E., Iliffe, S. and Davey, B. (2004) Social Work, General Practice and Evidence-based Policy in the Collaborative Care of Older People: Current Problems and Future Possibilities, *Health and Social Care in the Community* 12: 134–141

Kibble, D., Hamdi, N. and al Shuker, A. (2001) Young People in Britain and Jordan A Comparison of Religious Belief between East and West, *Theology* 104, 821: 335–344

Kolb, D. and associates (1994) *When Talk Works: Profiles of Mediators*, San Francisco, Jossey-Bass Publishers

Krebs, V. and Holley, J. (2006) *Building Smart Communities through Network Weaving* www.orgnet.com/Building Networks.pdf, accessed October 15 2006

Kubisch, A., Weiss, C., Schorr, L. and Connell, J. (1995) *New Approaches to Evaluating Community Initiatives: Concepts, Methods and Contexts*, Washington DC, The Aspen Institute

Laurent, C. (2005) Work in Progress, *Community Care*. 6–12 January

Laverack, G. and Labonte, R. (2000) A Planning Framework for Community Empowerment Goals within Health Promotion, *Health Policy and Planning* 15: 255–262

Leadbetter, C. (2004) *Personalisation through Participation*, London, Demos

LeCuyer-Maus, E. (2003) Stress and Coping in High-Risk Mothers: Difficult Life Circumstances, Psychiatric-Mental Health Symptoms, Education, and Experiences in Their Families of Origin, *Public Health Nursing* 30: 132–145

Ledwith, M. (2005) *Community Development*, Bristol, Policy Press

Lennon, B. (2004) *Peace Comes Dropping Slow: Dialogue and Conflict Management in Northern Ireland*, Belfast, Community Dialogue

Leventhal, T. and Brooks-Gunn, J. (2000) The Neighbourhoods They Live in: The Effects of Neighborhood Residence on Child and Adolescent Outcomes, *Psychological Bulletin* 126: 309–337

Linden, R. (2002) *Working Across Boundaries: Making Collaboration Work in Government and Nonprofit Organizations*, San Francisco, Jossey-Bass

Lipsky, M. (1980) *Street-Level Bureaucracy: Dilemmas of the Individual in Public Services*, New York, Russell Sage Foundation

Little, M. and Mount, K. (1999) *Prevention and Early Intervention with Children in Need*, Aldershot, Ashgate

Lloyd, N., O'Brien, M. and Lewis, C. (2003) *Fathers in Sure Start Local Programmes*, London, National Evaluation of Sure Start

Lloyd, N., O'Brien, M. and Lewis, C. (2002) *Underachieving Young Men Preparing for Work: A Report for Practitioners*, York, York Publishing Services

Local Government Association (2004) *Community Cohesion: An Action Guide*, London, LGA

Local Government Association and Association of Directors of Social Service (2003) *All Our Tomorrows: Inverting the Triangle of Care*, LGA and ADSS

London West Learning and Skills Council (2005) *Championing Family Learning: A Strategy for Family Learning in the London West Area*, London, LWLSC

Longley, C. (2006) I doubt if the law of blasphemy is worth saving, *The Tablet*, 18 February

Lynam, D., Wikstrom, P-O., Caspi A., Moffit, T., Loeber R. and Novak, S. (2000) The Interaction Between Impulsivity and Neighborhood Context on Offending: The Effects of Impulsivity are Stronger in Poorer Neighborhoods, *Journal of Abnormal Pyschology* 109: 563–574

Macpherson, Sir William (1999) *The Stephen Lawrence Enquiry* Cm 4262-1, London, TSO

Maddock, S. (2000) Managing the Development of Partnerships in Health Action Zones, *International Journal of Health Care Quality Assurance* 13: 65–73

Mann, P., Pritchard, S. and Rummery, K. (2004) Supporting Interorganizational Partnerships in the Public Sector, *Public Management Review* 6: 417–440

Margolin, L. (1997) *Under the Cover of Kindness: The Invention of Social Work*, Richmond, VA, University of Virginia Press

Markus, G. (2002) *Civic Participation in American Cities*, University of Michigan, Institute for Social Research

Martin, A. and Sanders, M. (2003) Balancing Work and Family: A Controlled Evaluation of the Triple P as a Work-site Intervention, *Child and Adolescent Mental Health* 8: 161–169

Martin, G., Nancarro, S., Parker, H., Phelps, K. and Regen, E. (2005) Place, Policy and Practitioners: On Rehabilitation, Independence and the Therapeutic Landscape in the Changing Geography of Care Provision to Older People in the UK, *Social Science and Medicine* 61: 1893–1904

Maxwell, D., Sodha, S. and Stanley, K. (2006) *An Asset Account for Looked After Children: A Proposal to Improve Educational Outcomes for Children in Care*, London, Institute for Public Policy Research

McGhee, D. (2003) Moving to 'Our' Common Ground – A Critical Examination of Community Cohesion Discourse in Twenty-first Century Britain, *The Sociological Review* 51: 376–404

Meijs, L. and Hoogstad, E. (2001) New Ways of Managing Volunteers: Combining Membership Management and Programme Management, *Voluntary Action* 3: 41–62

Melhuish, E. (2005) Early Impact of Sure Start Local Programmes on Children and Families, London, TSO

Millie, A., Jacobson, J., McDonald, E. and Hough, M. (2005) *Anti-Social Behaviour Strategies: Finding a Balance*, Bristol, Policy Press

Mittelmark, M. (1999) Health Promotion at the Communitywide Level, in N. Bracht (ed), *Health Promotion at the Community Level: New Advances*, London, Sage

Mollenkopf, J., Waters, M., Holdaway, J. and Kasinitz, P. (2005) The Ever-Winding Path: Ethnic and Racial Diversity in the Transition to Adulthood, in R. F. Settersten, F. Rumbaut, R. (eds), *On the Frontier of Adulthood: Theory, Research and Public Policy*, Chicago, University of Chicago Press

Moran, D., Ghate, D. and van der Merwe, A. (2004) *What Works in Parenting Support: A Review of International Evidence*, London, Department for Education and Skills

Morenoff, J., Sampson, R. and Raudenbush, W. (2001) Neighborhood Inequality, Collective Efficacy, and the Spatial dynamics of Urban Violence, *Criminology* 39, 3: 517–558

Morgan, R. (2006) *Young People's Views on Leaving Care*, London, Commission for Social Care Inspection

Morris, J., Blane, D. and White, I. (1996) Levels of Mortality, Education and Social Conditions in the 107 Local Education Authority Areas of England, *Journal of Epidemiology and Community Health* 50: 15–17

Mulgan, G. and Bury, F. (2006) *Double Devolution: The Renewal of Local Government*, London, The Young Foundation and John Smith Institute

Mullender, A. and Ward, D. (1991) *Self-Directed Groupwork: Users Take Action for Empowerment*, London, Whiting and Burch

Mulroy, E., Nelson, K. and Gour, D. (2005) Community Building and Family-Centred Service Collaboratives, *in* M. Weil (ed), *The Handbook of Community Practice*, London, Sage Publications

Murray, C. (1994) *Underclass: The Crisis Deepens*, London, Institute of Economic Affairs Health and Welfare Unit

Nacro (1999) *Youth Offending and Health: the role of YOTs*, London, Nacro

National Electronic Library for Health (2005) *Social Network Analysis*, London, NeLH

Neighbourhood renewal unit (2001) *A New Commitment to Neighbourhood Renewal: A National Strategy Action Plan*, London, Office of the Deputy Prime Minister

—— (2002a) *Floor Target Definitions*, London, Office of the Deputy Prime Minister

—— (2002b) *Reducing Re-offending in Ex-prisoners*, London, Office of the Deputy Prime Minister

—— (2005) *Neighbourhood Renewal Unit Race Equality Action Plan 2005*, London, Office of the Deputy Prime Minister

Netten, A., Forder, J. and Shapiro, J. (2006) *Measuring Personal Social Service Outputs for National Accounts: Services for Older People*, Manchester, Personal Social Services Research Unit

Niebuhr, R. (1932) *The Contribution of Religion to Social Work*, New York, Columbia University Press

Niskanen, W. (1971) *Bureaucracy and Representative Government*, New York, Aldine Atherton

Noor, A. (2000) Outlining Social Justice from an Islamic Perspective: An exploration, *Islamic Quarterly* 44, 2: 435–450

Office of the Deputy Prime Minister and Home Office (2005) *Citizen Engagement and Public Services: Why Neighbourhoods Matter*, London, ODPM

Office of the Deputy Prime Minister (2004) *The English Indices of Deprivation*, London, ODPM

—— (2005) *Local Area Agreements Guidance*, London, ODPM

—— (2006) *A Sure Start to Later Life: Ending Inequalities for Older People*, London, ODPM

Ousley, H. (2001) *Community Pride, Not Prejudice*, Bradford, Bradford City Council

Overman, H. (2002) Neighbourhood Effects in Large and Small Neighbourhoods, *Urban Studies* 39, 1: 117–130

Park, J. and Smith, C. (2000) 'To Whom Much Has Been Given . . .': Religious Capital and Community Voluntarism Among Churchgoing Protestants, *Journal of Scientific Study of Religion* 39, 3: 272–286

Patterson, G. (1992) *Anti-social Boys*, Eugene Oregon, Castalia Publishing Company

Patterson, G., Dishion, T. and Yoerger, K. (2000) Adolescent Growth in New Forms of Problem Behavior: Macro- and Micro-peer Dynamics, *Prevention Science* 1: 3–13

Patterson, O. (2006) A Poverty of Mind, *New York Times*, March 23

Paulo and the Community Work Forum (2003) *National Occupational Standards for Community Development Work*, London, Federation of Community Work Training Groups

Peach, C. (1996) Does Britain have Ghettos? *Transactions Institute of British Geographers* 21, 1: 216–235

Pearce, J. (2003) *Lessons from Northern Ireland: The Key Findings*, Presentation at Conference *Community Cohesion – Moving Bradford Forward: Lessons from Northern Ireland*, Bradford, City Hall

Pierson, J., Ing, P. and Gilford, S. (2004) *Making A Difference Evaluation of Blurton Sure Start*, Stoke on Trent, Housing and Community Research Unit, Staffordshire University

Pierson, J. and Gill, S. (2005) Believing and Belonging, in *Community, Work and Family: International Conference Proceedings*, Manchester, UK: 50–62

Pitcher, J., Campbell, R., Hubbard, P., O'Neill, M. and Scoular, J. (2006) *Living and Working in Areas of Street Sex Work: From Conflict to Coexistence*, Bristol, The Policy Press

Policy Action Team 4 (2000) *Neighbourhood Management*, London, Cabinet Office

Policy Action team 6 (2000) *Neighbourhood Wardens*, London, Cabinet Office

Policy Action Team 18 (2000) *Better Information*, London, Cabinet Office

Portes, A. (2003) Ethnicities: Children of Migrants in America, *Development* 46: 42–52

Power, A. (1997) *Estates on the Edge*, Basingstoke, Macmillan

Power, A. and Bergin, E. (1999) *Neighbourhood Management*, CASEpaper 31 London, Centre for Analysis of Social Exclusion, London School of Economics

Power, A. and Tunstall, R. (1996) *Swimming Against the Tide*, York, Joseph Rowntree Foundation

Pritchard, C. (2001) The Pyschosocial Impact of Child Abuse: Rediscovering the Poverty and Psychiatric Dimensions, *Primary Care Psychiatry* 7: 31–38

Provan, K. and Milward, H.B. (2001) Do Networks Really Work? A Framework for Evaluating Public-Sector Organizational networks, *Public Administration Review* 61, 4: 414–423

Pugh, G. and Statham, J. (2006) Interventions in Schools in the UK *in* McAuley, C., Pecora, P. and Rose, W. *Enhancing the Well-being of Children and Families through Effective Interventions: International Evidence for Practice*, London, Jessica Kingsley Publishers

Putnam, R. (2000) *Bowling Alone The Collapse and Revival of American Community*, London, Simon and Schuster

Radford, K., Hamilton, J. and Jarman, N. (2005) 'It's their word against mine': Young People's Attitudes to the Police Complaints Procedure in Northern Ireland, *Children and Society* 19: 360

Rankin, J. (2005) *A Mature Policy on Choice*, London, Institute of Public Policy Research

Rasmussen, K. and Smidt, S. (2003) Children in the Neighbourhood: The Neighbourhood in Children, in Christensen, P. and O'Brien, M. (eds), *Children in the City: Home, Neighbourhood and Community*, London, RoutledgeFalmer

Ray, R. and Street, A. (2005) Ecomapping: An Innovative Research Tool for Nurses, *Journal of Advanced Nursing* 50: 545–552

Resources for Change (2006) *Greater Chesterton Neighbourhood Action Planning Project Discussion Paper*, Newcastle under Lyme

Reynolds, L. (2006) Community Forums in Norwich, Personal communication to author

Roberts, J. (2004) *Alliances, Coalitions and Partnerships Building Collaborative Organizations*, Canada, New Society Publishers, Gabriola Island, BC

Rose, N. (2000) 'Community, Citizenship and the Third Way', *American Behavioural Scientist* 43, 9: 1395–1411

Rutter, M., Giller, H. and Hagell, A. (1998) *Anti-Social Behaviour by Young People*, Cambridge, Cambridge University Press

Ryan, S., Wiles, D., Cash, S. and Siebert, C. (2005) Risk Assessments: Empirically supported or values driven? *Children and Youth Services Review* 27: 213–225

Sabel, C. (1993) Studied Trust: Building New Forms of Cooperation in a Volatile Economy, *Human Relations* 46: 1133–1170

Safer Stronger Community Fund (2005) *Stronger Safer Communities: Implementation Guidance*, London, Home Office and Office of the Deputy Prime Minister

Saldanha, C. and Whittle, J. (1998) *Using the Logical Framework for Sector Analysis and Project Design*, Manila, Asian Development Bank

Sampson, R. (1999) What 'Community' Supplies, in R. A. D. Ferguson, W. (eds), *Urban Problems and Community Development*. Washington DC, Brookings Institution

Sampson, R., Morenoff, J. and Gannon-Rowley (2002) Assessing 'Neighborhood Effects': Social Processes and New Directions in Research, *Annual Review of Sociology* 28: 443–478

Sampson, R., Raudenbush, S. and Earls, F. (1997) Neighborhoods and Violent Crime: A Multilevel Study of Collective Efficacy, *Science* 277: 918–924

Satymurti, C. (1981) *Occupational Survival: The Case of the Local Authority Social Worker*, Oxford, Blackwell

Scharf, T. (2002) *Growing Older in Socially Deprived Areas: Social Exclusion in Later Life*, London, Help the Aged

Scharf, T., Phillipson, C. and Smith, E. (2005) *Multiple Exclusion and Quality of Life amongst Excluded Older People in Disadvantaged Neighbourhoods*, London, ODPM

Schier, S. (2000) *By Invitation Only: The Rise of Exclusive Politics in the United States*, Pittsburgh, University of Pittsburgh Press

Schwartz, B. (2004) *The Paradox of Choice: Why More is Less*, New York, HarperCollins

Schweinart, L. and Weikart, D. (1997) The High/Scope Preschool Curriculum Comparison Study Through Age 23, *Early Childhood Research Quarterly* 12: 117–143

Scott, J. (1998) *Seeing Like a State: How Certain Schemes to Improve the Human Condition Have Failed*, New Haven, Yale University Press

Scottish Executive (2005) *Determined to Succeed and Young People at Risk*, Edinburgh, Scottish Executive

Scottish Executive (2006) *Changing Lives Review of Social Work in the 21st Century*, Edinburgh, Scottish Executive

Seaman, P., Turner, K., Hill, M., Stafford, A. and Walker, M. (2006) *Parenting and Children's Resilience in Disadvantaged Communities*, London, National Children's Bureau in association with the Joseph Rowntree Foundation

Settersten, R. (2005) Social Policy and the Transition to Adulthood, in Settersten, R., Furstenberg, F. and Rumbaut, R. (eds) 2005. *On the Frontier of Adulthood Theory, Research, and Public Policy*, Chicago, The University of Chicago Press

Settersten, R., Furstenberg, F. and Rumbaut, R. (eds) (2005) *On the Frontier of Adulthood Theory, Research, and Public Policy*, Chicago, The University of Chicago Press

Shonkoff, J. and Phillips, D. (eds) (2001) *From Neurons to Neighborhoods: The Science of Early Childhood Development*, Washington, DC, National Academy Press

Shumov, L., Vandell, D. and Posner, J. (1999) Risk and Resilience in the Urban Neighborhood: Predictors of Academic Performance Among Low-income Elementary School Children, *Merrill-Palmer Quarterly* 45: 309–331

Shupe, A. and Misztal, B. eds (1998) *Religion, Mobilization and Social Action*, London, Praeger

Sleeter, C. and McLaren, P. (eds) (1995) *Multicultural Education, Critical Pedagogy and the Politics of Difference*, Albany, State University of New York Press

Smith, G. and Khanom, A. (2005) *Children's Perspectives on Believing and Belonging*, Findings, 0375 July, York, Joseph Rowntree Foundation

Smith, M. (2005) Health Warning, *Community Care*, 16–22 June

Snyder, W., Wenger, E. and Briggs, X. (2004) Communities of Practice in Government: Leveraging Knowledge for Performance, *The Public Manager* 32: 17–22

Social Exclusion Unit (2003) *A Better Education for Children in Care*, London, Cabinet Office

Specht, H. and Courtney, M. (1994) *Unfaithful Angels: How Social Work Has Abandoned its Mission*, New York, The Free Press

Stoke on Trent (2005) *Neighbourhood Statistics*, Stoke on Trent, Knowledge Management Unit

Strack, R., Magill, C. and McDonagh, K. (2004) Engaging Youth Through Photovoice, *Health Promotion Practice* 5: 49–58

Thomas, J. (1995) *Public Participation in Public Decisions: New Skills and Strategies for Public Managers*, San Francisco, Jossey-Bass

Thompson, J. (2002) *Community Education and Neighbourhood Renewal*, Leicester, National Institute of Adult Continuing Education

United Nations (1995) *Human Development Report: Gender and Human Development*, New York, UN

Utting, D., Rose, W. and Pugh, G. (2002) *Better Results for Children and Families. Involving Communities in Planning Services Based on Outcomes*, London, NCVCCO

van Tilburg, W. (1998) Losing and Gaining in Old Age: Changes in Personal Network Size and Social Support in a Four-Year Longitudinal Study, *Journal of Gerontology Series B: Psychological Sciences and Social Sciences* 53, 6: S313–S323

Verba, S., Schlozman, K. and Brady, H. (1995) *Voice and Equality: Civic Voluntarism in American Politics*, Cambridge, Mass, Harvard University Press

Waldfogel, J. (2005) Social Mobility, Life Chances and the Early Years, in Delorenzi, S., Reed,

J. and Robinson, P. (eds) *Maintaining Momentum: Promoting Social Mobility and Life Chances from Early Years to Adulthood*, London, Institute of Public Policy Research

Warwick, I., Aggleton, P., Chase, E., Schagen, S., Blenkinsop, S., Schagen, I., Scott, E. and Eggers, M. (2005) Evaluating Healthy Schools: Perceptions of Impact Among School-based Responsdents, *Health Education Research Theory and Practice* 20: 697–708

Webster-Stratton, C. (1992) *The Incredible Years: A Trouble Shooting Guide for Parents*, Toronto, Umbrella Press

Weil, M., Gamble, D. (2005) Evolution, Models, and the Changing Context of Community Practice, in M. Weil (ed), *The Handbook of Community Practice*, CA and London, Sage, Thousand Oaks

Wenger, C. (1997) Social Networks and the Prediction of Elderly People at Risk, *Aging and Mental Health* 1: 311–320

Wenger, C., Davies, R., Shahtahmasebi, S. and Scott, A. (1996) Social Isolation and Loneliness in Old Age: Review and Model Refinement, *Ageing and Society* 16: 333–358

Wenger, E. (1998) *Communities of Practice: Learning, Meaning, and Identity*, Cambridge, Cambridge University Press

Werbner, P. (2005) *The Translocation of Culture: Migration, Community and the Force of Multiculturalism in History*, Paper 48 IIIS, Dublin, Institute for International Integration Studies

Whelan, J., Swallow, M., Peschar, P. and Dunne, A. (2002) From Counselling to Community Work: Developing a Framework for Social Practice, *Australian Social Work* 55: 13–23

White, S. and Featherstone, B. (2005) Communicating Misunderstandings: Multi-agency Work as Social Practice, *Child and Family Social Work* 10: 207–216

Wikstrom, P. and Loeber, R. (2000) Do Disadvantaged Neighborhoods Cause Well-adjusted Children to Become Adolescent Delinquents? A Study of Male Juvenile Serious Offending, Individual Risk and Protective Factors and Neighborhood Context, *Criminology* 38, 4: 1109–1142

Wilkinson, R. (1996) *Unhealthy Societies The Affliction of Inequality*, London, Routledge

Williams, R. (2005) *Who's bringing up our children?* Citizen Organising Foundation lecture, University of London, Queen Mary College

Wilson, M. and Wilde, M. (2003) *Benchmarking Community Participation: Developing and Implementing the Active Partners Benchmarks*, York, Joseph Rowntree Foundation

Wilson, W. (1987) *The Truly Disadvantaged*, Chicago, University of Chicago Press

—— (1996) *When Work Disappears*, New York, Alfred A. Knopf

Woolhead, G., Calnan, M., Dikeppe, P. and Tadd, W. (2004) Dignity in Older Age: What Do Older People in the United Kingdom Think? *Age and Ageing* 33: 165–170

Worley, C. (2005) 'It's not about race. It's about the community': New Labour and 'community cohesion', *Critical Social Policy* 25, 4: 483–496

Wuthnow, R. (2002) Religious Involvement and Status-Bridging Social Capital, *Journal for the Scientific Study of Religion* 41, 4: 669–684

Wymer, W. and Starness, B. (2001) Conceptual Foundations and Practical Guidelines for Recruiting Volunteers to Serve in Local Nonprofit Organisations, *Journal of Nonprofit and Public Sector Marketing* 9: 63–96

Yorkshire Forward (2000) *Active Partners: Benchmarking Community Participation in Regeneration*, Leeds, Yorkshire Forward

Young, J., Robinson, M., Chell, S., Sanderson, D., Chaplin, S., Burns, E. and Fear, J. (2005) A Prospective Baseline Study of Frail Older People Before the Introduction of an Intermediate Care Service, *Health and Social Care in the Community* 13, 4: 307–312

Young, M. and Willmott, P. (1963) *Family and Kinship in East London*, London, Pelican

Youth Justice Board (2006) *Suitable, Sustainable, Supported: A Strategy to Ensure Provision of Accommodation for Children and Young People Who Offend*, London, Youth Justice Board

—— 2007 *Accommodation: Needs and Experiences* London, YJB

INDEX